THE ESSENTIAL MIXOLOGIST™

22 Original Essential Oil Infused Recipes

WRITING AND ORIGINAL RECIPES
JULEZ WEINBERG

PHOTOGRAPHS
JULEZ WEINBERG

DESIGN & LAYOUT
NAILIA MINNEBAEVA

The "What is an Essential Oil" section, "The dōTERRA® difference" section, "Co-Impact Sourcing®" section and all the additional information about each essential oil provided under the recipes is information courtesy of doterra.com

For more information on any of these subjects please visit doterra.com

National Library of USA Cataloguing-in-Publication data:

ISBN: 978-0-692-99041-4

www.marketingmentor.live (design by Nailia Minnebaeva)

DISCLAIMER:

This book has been created with the intention to provide information to help educate the reader in regard to the subject matter covered. It is sold with the understanding that the author is not liable for the misconception, misunderstanding and misuse of any of the information provided. The information in this book is not provided with the intention to diagnose, prescribe, or treat any disease, illness or injured condition of the body. The author of this book shall have neither liability or responsibility to any person or entity with respect to any loss, damage, or injury caused, or allegedly to be caused, directly or indirectly by the information contained within this book. The information provided in this book is in no way intended as a substitute for professional medical counseling. Anyone suffering from any disease, illness, or injury should consult a qualified health professional.

DEDICATION

This book is dedicated to my late father, Michael Weinberg. Somehow, from the other side — from a place where I cannot see you, but can certainly feel you-you have encouraged and supported me to step into my passion and share this part of myself with the world. It's been said that cardinals are a sign there's a visitor from heaven. A cardinal has been present for most of my photo shoots for this book. I have also heard him chirping while my fingers tap the keys as I am writing, as though we have been collaborating on a beautiful song together. In fact, he is singing outside my window right now. Thank you for being a presence during this creation. I love you always, poppy.

GRATITUDE

I will first express my deepest gratitude to whom many refer to as God, and whom others call the All Mighty Presence, Great Spirit, Divine Mother, Divine Father, Buddha, Krishna, Jesus, Mary, Allah, Yahweh: there are so many other wonderful ways we address the All That Is. Thank you for your eternal presence in my life. Thank you for helping me to be a vessel of creative expression, love and beauty in the world. I am ever so grateful to you and humbled by you.

I begin my journey of gratitude with my love, my dearest friend, my amazing business partner and precious spouse, Meredith Kelly. I am the luckiest girl on the planet to be supported by you in this life. Thank you for always encouraging me to share my gifts with the world. Thank you for being a constant source of inspiration. Thank you for being the number one taste-tester for all of my crazy concoctions. Thank you for always believing in me, even when I had lost my way and didn't believe in myself. Thank you for being the one to gently guide me back into the world of aromatic plants and the gift of essential oils. Thank you for not only being my muse, but for also actually contributing your beautiful gifts and talents to the photo shoot for this book. Your ethereal essence and magical eye for beauty made this book even more magnificent. I love you with all my heart and feel excited and inspired to continue creating with you in this lifetime.

I would like to express my deep gratitude to Nailia Minnebaeva. It has been an honor and a joy to work in tandem with you on the layout and design of this book. Your spirit and design sensibility unveiled the essence of my vision beyond what I imagined on my own. Thank you.

I would like to express my deep gratitude to the founding executives at dōTERRA® — Emily Wright, Dave Sterling, Dr. David Hill, Corey Lindley, Rob Young, Gregory Cook, and Mark Wolfert — for creating a company with the integrity and standards which allow for complete and total freedom to bring these essential oil-infused recipes to life. Because of your dedication and commitment to quality, the world gets to experience these gifts of the earth every day, and I am completely grateful to each of you for this. Thank you.

To Marnie Harrison, I am utterly grateful to you for introducing us to dōTERRA®. Thank you for your patience and support. You brought us both something that has changed our lives forever.

I would like to thank the farmers who grow these beautiful aromatic plants, and all of the people who are involved from seed to bottle. It takes a lot of time and dedication to create an essential oil. Thank you for all of your hard work and commitment to making sure we get the best essential oils on the planet. I am truly grateful for all that you do to ensure this process and the end results.

I would like to thank our dōTERRA® team, Team Cultivate Wellness. You all amaze me each and every day with your passion for sharing these beautiful oils with the world. Your support and love for The Essential Mixologist body of work has been a joy and a blessing. I love receiving texts from so many of you asking for different recipes, and I am excited that you will now have a reference at your fingertips. I am grateful for each and every one of you.

I would like to thank my colleague Angela Hager for all of her love, support and excitement around The Essential Mixologist. You have been a cheerleader of this work from the beginning, and I am grateful for the space you have provided in the past to showcase these concoctions to your (our) team. I truly appreciate everything you do to move your business along and to continue sharing this mission with the world. Thank you!

I would like to thank many of my friends (too many to mention) and family for always encouraging my creations, and for enjoying them each time I have had the honor of mixing something special for you. You know who you are: we have shared a cocktail or two, and I'm always grateful for our time together.

To my mother, Sheila, thank you for sharing your love for creating things in the kitchen with me at an early age and for always believing in me. I love you.

To my sister, Barri, thank you for always believing in me and for thinking of ways to help me share my message with the world. I love you.

To my mother-in-law, Cyndi, thank you for encouraging me over the years to put out a recipe book. I finally followed your gentle guidance, and I know it will be the first of many. I love you.

To Kerri Ialongo-Gillette, thank you for recognizing the plant medicine woman and alchemist living within me, and for inviting me to open Herbalicious with you. It changed my life in so many ways, fortified my connection to the plant kingdom and created a place for the love of my life to find me. I am so totally grateful for your presence in my life.

To Holly, Jarred and Eli Matteson, thank you for your support and excitement around this body of work. I am grateful I had the opportunity to turn your amazing kitchen into my own personal test kitchen, and for Eli's willingness to be my little assistant alchemist.

To Jane Harper and Christie Hardwick, thank you for your support and love of my alchemy. You have been a consistent cheerleader of The Essential Mixologist and have opened your home on many occasions for me to share these recipes with your community. I am grateful to both of you.

To Jennifer Smira, I am so grateful to have you as a part of my life journey. You provided the space for my first creation, and if it wasn't for your friendship and presence in my life, who knows if this inspiration would have ever come to fruition. Thank you.

To Daryn Payne, thank you for being a testament to; "When the student is ready, the teacher will appear." Your timely presence in my life assisted my inner alchemist to take full flight. You will always hold a place in my heart.

To Lissy Dickens, thank you for being such a beautiful presence and connector in my aromatic plant journey. I will never forget seeing your smiling face at Expo East and knowing with certainty, I had found an old friend. I trust you are frolicking freely in that big lavender field in the sky - laughing about just how perfect it all really is. I miss you, my sweet friend.

To Caryn Gehlmann, thank you for being a part of my life and my journey with essential oils. It would be incomplete not to acknowledge our connection through the aromatic plant kingdom and the important role you once played there for me, and continue to play for many others. I have a deep respect and admiration for you. Our time together will always hold a special place in my heart.

To Bryna Rene Haynes, thank you for being a source of information to guide me through my first book venture. I am so grateful for the quickly answered texts and time you took to walk me through so many unknowns. It looks like the "Teahouse" gave birth to a couple of authors indeed.

I want to express the gratitude I have for Provincetown - I am so blessed to live here. Artists come from all over the world to drink from this well of creativity. It has been a dream for many years to live in this magical village by the sea. It recently dawned on me how amazing it is that I got to give birth to this book in a place that inspires so many. Thank you, Provincetown. Thank you for your love. Thank you for allowing me to make my home here. Thank you for your light.

Lastly, I would like to directly thank the aromatic plants and the essential oils themselves. You are all like dear friends with distinct personalities, properties and of course, signature aromas. I know you are a living, breathing life-force on this planet and the world needs you now more than ever. I am in complete awe of your magic and in total gratitude for your presence on the earth and in my life. Thank you, thank you, thank you.

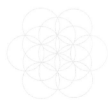

"LET FOOD BE THY MEDICINE
AND MEDICINE BE THY FOOD".

– HIPPOCRATES

HIGHLIGHTS

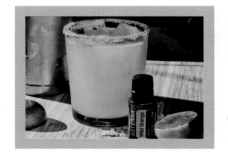
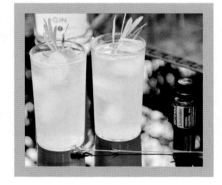
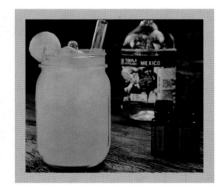
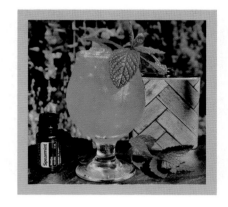
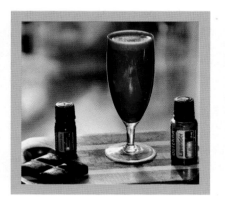
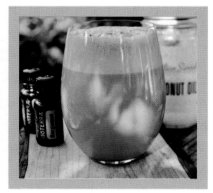

CONTENTS

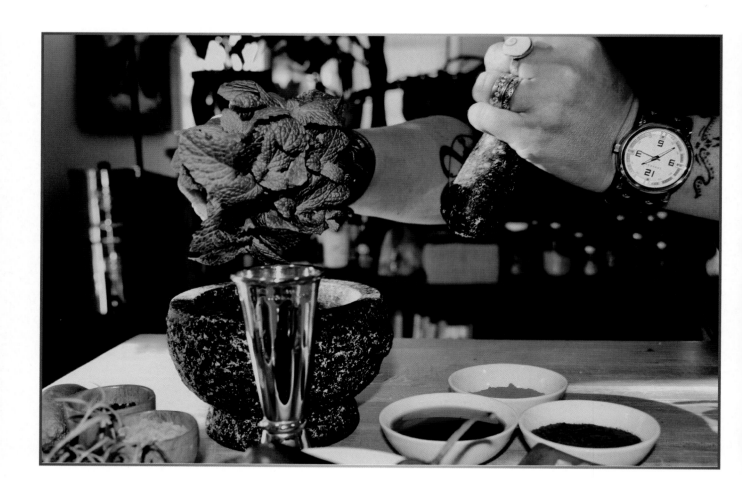

SALUTATIONS

I've always considered myself a purist at heart: I love items that are homegrown and scratch made. I appreciate the process of things, especially when it comes to food and drink. My palate doesn't like to be overstimulated by synthetic and contrived flavors or lackluster processed ingredients. I'm interested in the taste of real fruits, vegetables, plants, flowers, roots, and herbs. I believe many of us have lost our awareness of these magical ingredients, and in our poor attempt to create a replacement for what nature has already provided, we have created a synthetic cacophony of toxicity.

My philosophy is not unique. I would say I'm part of a growing movement that encourages the use of ingredients in their purest forms, and the craft creation of as much of what we put into our bodies as is possible. I'm a farm-to-table, pier-to-plate, locavore, slow food, organic, non-GMO, artisan, curated, craft cocktail kind of girl. There, I said it. Now, let's talk about what this book is really about.

The Essential Mixologist is about the art of maximizing flavor and weaving medicinal ingredients into cocktails through the use of essential oils to create aromatic elixirs. In any one of these recipes, the alcohol component can easily be omitted to create a mocktail. A simple definition of an elixir is a magic and medicinal potion. Therefore, each of these 22 recipes is, without question, an elixir — with or without the alcohol.

I recognize there is a world of shrubs and bitters included in most craft cocktail recipes. Let me say that I absolutely love these ingredients and use them all the time.

However, this book is based on a different approach. My method here maximizes flavor through the simplicity of essential oils while adding medicinal elements to cocktails. I'm not a renowned mixologist (yet), and this book is not about me waving around my titles or credentials. I'm just a girl who loves to create with nature. Throughout my journey, I have cultivated a bible of recipes that have captivated the palates of hundreds of people — enough to finally encourage me to write this book and share it with the world.

I encourage you to get familiar with the information I provide about each of the essential oils being used in these recipes. I would love for every reader to be aware that each time you imbibe one of these elixirs, you are opening yourself up to a world of flavor, an aromatic feast of the senses and most importantly, an array of beautiful, natural solutions from the plant kingdom to support your body, mind, and spirit.

The Essential Mixologist is an invitation to your inner alchemist — an invitation to play and to create the most amazing cocktails with health-enhancing properties right from the comfort of your home. It's a book about embracing the art of mixology and the simplicity of sharing not just a cocktail with friends, but rather a medicinal cocktail with friends.

Enjoy the journey and cheers!

Always with love, Julez.

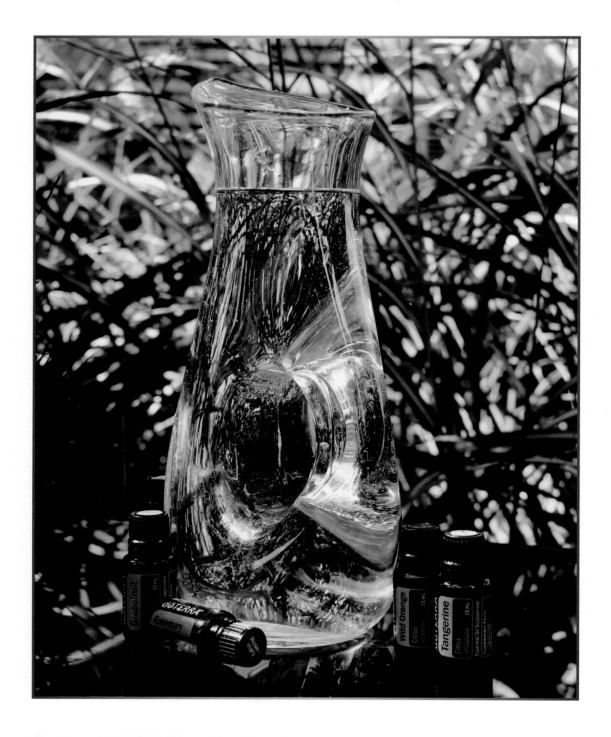

AN ALCHEMIST IS BORN

I'm a tree hugger, and I recognized the symbiotic relationship between plants and humans at a very early age. Let's look at the facts: plants are part of a complex process where the by-product is oxygen. The last time I checked, us humans need oxygen to stay alive. Because plants play this important role in sustaining our life-force, I would say they are definitely our allies and even our friends. Plants create so much for us: food for us to eat; medicine that can heal our bodies, minds, and spirits; and various other useful commodities. They also create beauty all around us in the form of vivid colors. Some plants — the aromatic plant kingdom specifically — create essential oils, which are the focus of this book.

I'll share a little secret with you. It might sound crazy, but it truly happened to me: I had a real-life exchange with a forest of plants. To translate: all of the plants around me communicated with me. It was actually one of several communications I have had with the plant kingdom, and it changed my life.

When I was in my early-to-mid-twenties, I was visiting friends in New Jersey. It was a beautiful late summer day, and I was lying in a hammock in the backyard. Everything was so alive: I could smell the fragrances of many different flowers, herbs, and trees as a slight breeze blew. In the distance, I heard laughter on the wind. It was so sweet and genuine that I began to laugh with it. As I laughed with the wind, a thought filled my mind. I heard, "Pay attention to us, we will be paying your bills." It sounds kooky, but it happened. I was instantly aware that it was a message from the plants, and I started laughing even louder. At that point, my friends yelled over and asked if everything was okay. I quickly pulled myself together and said I was fine, and that I had a funny memory come over me.

I laid back in that hammock for quite some time. I could feel the energy of the forest with all of its beauty pulsating around me. It was magical. I had no idea what it meant in the moment, but several months later, I was studying herbs. I had become co-owner in a health and wellness business where we provided herbal consultations along with other services and also sold herbal plant medicine in all forms.

It was here, at Herbalicious, where I met essential oils for the first time in this lifetime. It was truly love at first smell. I fell in love so deeply that at times I was brought to tears by my experiences with the essential oils. My connection with this wonderful and magical world of aromatic plants was strong: it was like meeting old friends again, and I immediately began channeling an inner alchemist who felt as though she had been lying dormant in me since forever. Discovering this part of myself, I was at home with my soul.

I soon attracted a teacher — a fellow alchemist. He taught me many things about blending essential oils and using them in a variety of ways to assist the body, mind and spirit. It was something I felt like I already intuitively understood, and my ability to create potions for myself and for others quickly moved

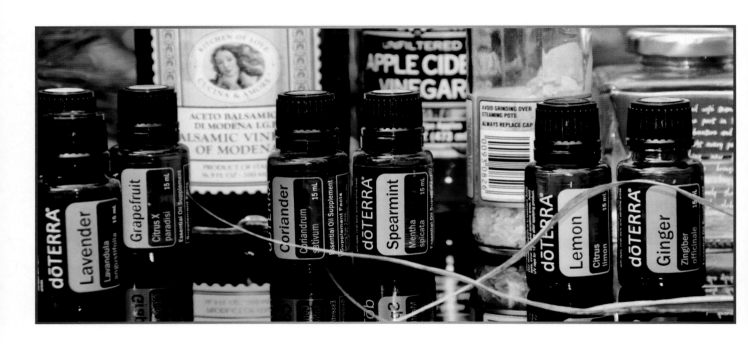

into action and expression. I even created a blending station in the cellar of Herbalicious. It was my own space to create magic and connect with the plants, and I learned a lot about them during that time.

One day, I was with my teacher; we were spending a weekend together with friends in Sarasota, Florida and learning more about the oils. We came to the end of our day, and I suggested we break for cocktails. I was a bartender throughout college and for years after: I liked the fun of it, and the extra cash. I had always enjoyed making drinks using unique ingredients. My teacher had brought some very special jasmine essential oil from a pure source, and I had fallen in love with the aroma and the energy of that plant. I asked if it would be okay for me to use a little to create a round of cocktails for us, and he agreed wholeheartedly that this would be a wonderful experiment.

This was the birthing moment where my alchemy was taken to a whole new level of expression, and my first aromatic cocktail was born: a jasmine spritzer. It was divine. We all felt like we were drinking the nectar of the Gods. It was beautiful and aromatic, and its effects on the psyche were amazing — we all felt relaxed and totally calm.

I began experimenting with high-grade essential oils I knew were from trusted sources. Over time, I created many recipes of unique essential oil-infused cocktails that became well-known where I lived. I started receiving invitations to experiment with these concoctions at parties, and I became known as a mixologist and alchemist. I even caught the attention of a local chef who loved my jasmine spritzer and used it for a concept dinner she created. She went on to be featured in Food & Wine Magazine, where she credited me for the creation of this essential oil-infused cocktail. Food & Wine called me to confirm the information and did a short interview with me. I'm actually mentioned in the article, my one claim to fame as a mixologist.

Over the years, life brought me back to my original career choice as a producer, and my sweetheart and I moved to the West Coast. I stayed connected to the essential oils; it seemed they followed me wherever I went. When I say they were always around me, I mean they were always around me. I used them personally and also continued to share them. They remained a constant in my life, like trusted friends that were there when I needed them.

Several years ago, life brought me full circle once again. My career as a producer had reached an exciting high point, and then suddenly imploded. Let's say it had something and everything to do the economy crashing and all investment capital coming to a screeching halt. Like so many others at that time, I found myself at a crossroads without any advance warning.

We wound up moving back to the East Coast. Shortly after the move, a dear friend sent a care package of essential oils from a company called dōTERRA®. I immediately knew when I opened a bottle that these oils were very different. I was familiar with quality and had been collecting the best essential oils I could find for many years at that point. However, these oils were on another level. They smelled crisper and they worked faster — they were superior in all ways. I was astounded by the quality. I began using them exactly as I had been using essential oils for many years and the results I got were better — in fact, they were 100%.

I started learning more about dōTERRA® and their CPTG® (certified pure, therapeutic grade) certification. I learned about what made these oils different, and I felt comfortable experimenting with internal usage with so many more oils than I had felt I could through my other resources. My entire world of alchemy through mixology began opening up, and I began getting really creative. I also opted to continue my education and became a certified health coach through The Institute for Integrative Nutrition.

In time, my wife Meredith and I chose dōTERRA® as our next venture and began building our own business. Our choice has proven to be extremely successful, and in three years' time, we are Blue Diamonds with the company and have teams around the world. I have been able to find true freedom as an alchemist and mixologist and have taken things to a whole new level with my creations.

As a health-minded person, I believe in balance. I like to socialize, and I like to have fun. There are many people who would object to the words "healthy" and "cocktails" being used in the same sentence, but I beg to differ. I believe cocktailing can be fun in moderation and even healthy with the added benefits of essentials oils. Using these beautiful CPTG® essential oils to concoct wonderful, delicious drinks with health benefits has been an absolute joy: an opportunity to share with people, and an outlet for my creative expression.

I believe that plants are here for many reasons and that they also want to come out and play with us in the world. They want to be a part of the conversation, at the dinner party as well as on the dance floor. Conscious cocktailing from a purist perspective, using only dōTTERA® CPTG® essential oils (because we know they are the best), is not only fun but is also actually good for you and good your soul.

I also want to say this for total and complete clarity: I am aware that consuming alcohol is not congruent for everyone. If alcohol isn't congruent with your chemistry or doesn't fit in with your spiritual beliefs, please don't dismiss these recipes. I encourage you to leave out the alcohol and mix yourself a delicious mocktail that will leave your taste buds soaring and your spirit enlivened. These recipes stand alone without alcohol. With the inclusion of the essential oils, they each have an array of beneficial properties and will wow your palate every time. There are many occasions where I leave out the alcohol and simply enjoy them as wonderful elixirs.

Lastly, if you choose to fully imbibe with these recipes, please choose to do so responsibly. My message isn't about intoxication. I have measurements for a reason. I endorse the timeless dance of sharing a cocktail with friends in moderation. Cocktails are meant to be sipped and savored — not guzzled. Please make a choice to imbibe responsibly. In addition, hydration matters. It's important when consuming a beverage containing alcohol to drink a lot of water. I recommend a few drops of lemon essential oil or any of the other citrus oils for flavor and support. I include suggestions for this in the book. Finally, please don't imbibe and drive. Be mindful of your consumption and act accordingly. Your life and the lives of others depend on your sensibility. When in doubt, Uber, Lyft or a good old-fashioned taxi cab are great choices.

I am so excited to introduce you to these 22 recipes. I should let you know this is only the beginning and The Essential Mixologist is the first of many creations I will be offering to you as my audience. I am so excited to begin this journey with you.

May the pages of this book open up your heart to the magic of the aromatic plant kingdom and to the gift of these essential oils. May you find their laughter in the wind and may it invite your own laughter to play, dance and imbibe with them in the most delicious ways!

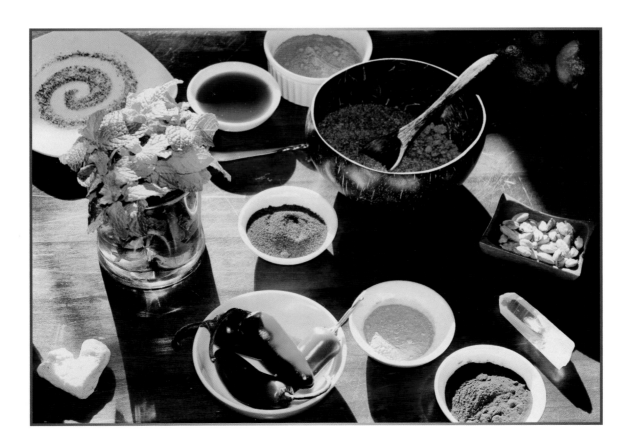

PERMISSION TO MODIFY

Please allow your creativity, needs and flavor desires to win every time. I have created these recipes because I feel they showcase the ingredients I have chosen in the best way possible for MY palate. We are all created bio-individually, and what I think tastes good may not taste good to another. What I think is sweet may not be sweet enough for another. Where I like tequila, someone else might prefer vodka and someone else might prefer no alcohol at all. Where I have said to use wild orange essential oil, someone else may prefer lime or grapefruit. If you are a recipe person and need to follow a recipe, I feel these won't let you down. However, a squirt of agave for me may be a longer squirt for you. I give you permission to modify, and I ask you to give yourself permission to modify. Make it how you like it, and know your inner alchemist also wants to play—allow it the space and freedom to do so.

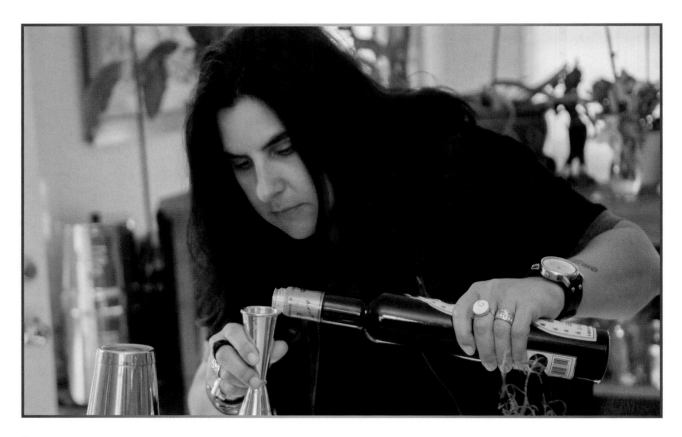

WHAT IS AN ESSENTIAL OIL?

If you have ever enjoyed the scent of a rose, you've experienced the aromatic qualities of essential oils. These naturally occurring, volatile aromatic compounds are found in the seeds, bark, stems, roots, flowers, and other parts of plants. They can be both beautifully and powerfully fragrant. Essential oils give plants their distinctive smells, essential oils protect plants and play a role in plant pollination. In addition to their intrinsic benefits to plants and their beautiful fragrance, essential oils have long been used for food preparation, beauty treatment, and health-care practices.

But what exactly is a volatile aromatic compound? In short, these compounds are small organic molecules that tend to change quickly from their solid or liquid state to a gas at room temperature. They are called volatile because they change state quickly. When you first open a bottle of essential oil, you instantly notice that the aroma is potent and you can smell it typically even from some distance. The physical and chemical properties of the volatile aromatic compounds that compose essential oils allow them to quickly move through the air and directly interact with the olfactory sensors in the nose. Such unique properties make essential oils ideal for applications inclusion in aromatherapy – using these compounds from plants to help maintain a healthy mind and body – as well as other applications. The type of volatile aromatic compounds present in an essential oil determines both the oil's aroma and the benefits it offers.

Over 3,000 varieties of volatile aromatic compounds have been identified to date. The nature of an essential oil varies from plant to plant, within botanical families, and from species to species. The delicate ratio of aromatic constituents found in any given essential oil are what make it unique and give it specific benefits.

Even with pure essential oils the composition of the oil can vary depending on the time of day, season, geographic location, method and duration of distillation, year grown, and the weather, making every step of the production process a critical determinant of the overall quality of the essential oil product.

Essential oils can be used for a wide range of emotional and physical wellness applications. They can be used as single essential oils or in complex essential oil blends depending on user experience and desired benefit.

In this book, we will be exploring a variety of drink recipes where we use essential oils as the primary flavor profile and simultaneously create health-promoting elixirs.

THE dōTERRA® DIFFERENCE

You are going to learn a lot of fun recipes from this book, and you will get excited about the creative flavors and their medicinal properties. Chances are you will be so excited that you will want to get some essential oils and begin playing immediately. Before we begin this journey, it's critical that I am clear about this very important truth: NOT ALL ESSENTIAL OILS ARE CREATED EQUAL. If you take away anything from this book, this would be the best thing I could offer you.

There's a reason why, after using essential oils for almost 20 years, I only use dōTERRA®. Here it is:

When you choose dōTERRA®, you are choosing essential oils gently and carefully distilled from plants that have been patiently harvested at the perfect moment by experienced growers from around the world for ideal extract composition and efficacy.

Each dōTERRA® essential oil is also carefully and thoroughly tested using the strict CPTG® Certified Pure Therapeutic Grade® quality protocol. Experienced essential oil users will immediately recognize the superior quality standard for naturally safe, purely effective therapeutic-grade dōTERRA® essential oils.

While there is a science to the distillation of essential oils, it is also an art. Distillers not only rely on years of experience, they also employ modern technologies and techniques.

The most common method of extracting essential oils is a low-heat steam distillation process. In this process, pressurized steam is circulated through plant material. The essential oils are liberated from the plant and carried away by the steam. When the steam cools, the water and oils naturally separate and the oil is collected. To ensure the highest quality oil extract with the correct chemical composition, the temperature and pressure must be closely monitored. Too little heat or pressure and the oil will not release; too much, and the oil's composition and potency will be affected.

STEAM DISTILLATION

Steam distillation is the most common way to extract aromatic compounds (essential oil) from a plant. During the steam distillation process, steam passes through the plant material. The combination of heated steam and gentle pressure causes the essential oil to be released from microscopic protective sacs. As the vapor mixture flows through a condenser and cools, it yields a layer of oil and a layer of water. The essential oil rises to the top and is separated from the hydrosol (floral water) and collected.

Some have asked about the difference between first distillations in comparison to complete distillations. The temperature for steam distilling is usually between 140–212 degrees Fahrenheit.

Since different plants require different pressures, times, and temperatures, using this particular distillation method makes it possible to adjust the temperature based on the plant type, making it a very effective and precise way to obtain the purest compounds.

EXPRESSION

Unlike steam distillation, expression, sometimes referred to as "cold pressed," does not involve heat. In this process, oil is extracted from the product under mechanical pressure. dōTERRA® uses expression to extract all of its citrus oils, such as Wild Orange, Lemon, Lime, Bergamot, and Grapefruit, from the rind.

Proper distillation requires a consideration for the uniqueness of pressure, temperature, time, and harvesting practices, each of which may be as diverse as the plants themselves. A poor distillation process can alter or destroy the necessary aromatic compounds that comprise the essential oil, leaving a substance far different from the intended goal and something that would not be used to support health and wellness. For this reason, the best distillation artisans dedicate their efforts and work to only a few select plants. This focused effort develops proper knowledge and experience, helping ensure congruency between the oil chemistry of the plant and its distilled form.

CPTG® QUALITY TESTING

The purity of an essential oil is its most important characteristic. An essential oil that isn't pure means you run the risk of putting germs, heavy metals, or adulterants onto or into your body, which can provoke irritation, adverse effects, or even sickness. Without an accepted standard for essential oil quality, dōTERRA® created its own testing process, calling it CPTG® Certified Pure Therapeutic Grade®. The CPTG® process certifies that there are no added fillers, synthetic ingredients, or harmful contaminants in their essential oils that would reduce their efficacy. dōTERRA® even goes a step further, putting all their products and the packaging through a battery of tests to ensure a long and effective shelf-life. This protocol ensures potency, purity, and consistency batch to batch.

BEFORE THE CPTG® PROCESS BEGINS

Proper methods of growing, harvesting, and distilling are also crucial to maintaining purity. Poor production practices and the development of synthetic essential oil variations suggest that it is impossible to accurately identify a pure essential oil without scientific analysis. Appropriate analysis of the constituents within an essential oil is one of the most challenging and detailed aspects of quality assurance.

Knowing which of the many different species of a given plant will provide the most profound therapeutic health benefits is the first step in producing the highest quality essential oil. Relying on the expertise of botanists, chemists and wellness practitioners, botanical materials are carefully selected for their natural concentrations of active aromatic compounds.

Nurturing plants in the most favorable environment and carefully harvesting and transporting plant material for processing ensures an optimal yield of pure and potent essential oils. Spanning the continents of the globe, dōTERRA's exclusive network of growers and harvesters are experts at cultivating plants specific to the essential oil industry.

THE CPTG® PROCESS

The CPTG® testing begins immediately after distillation with each oil being reviewed for its chemical composition. A second round of testing is carried out at our production facility to ensure that what was distilled and tested is the same essential oil as was received. A third review of the chemistry of the oil is conducted in a three-phase procedure as the oils are packaged into the bottles we use as consumers. Each of these tests confirms that the essential oil is free of contaminants and unexpected alterations during production.

The CPTG® Certified Pure Therapeutic Grade quality protocol includes the following tests:

- Organoleptic testing
- Microbial testing
- Gas chromatography
- Mass spectrometry
- Fourier Transform Infrared spectroscopy (FTIR)
- Chirality testing
- Isotopic analysis
- Heavy metal testing

Historically, gas chromatography was sufficient to identify individual components in an essential oil. However, as more sophisticated methods for developing synthetic essential oil products formed, further validation methods were needed. Over time, additional testing methods such as mass spectroscopy, chiral analysis, FTIR Scan, carbon isotope analysis and others have been developed to more accurately identify each individual essential oil constituent.

This may have been slightly more information then you require about essential oils. However, my appreciation for the perfection dōTERRA® supplies us with is something I felt could not be left out. If you had any questions about including these oils in recipes you will be consuming, I trust they have been answered and that confidence now prevails.

CO-IMPACT SOURCING®

Before we get started, the last significant piece of the dōTERRA® puzzle I will mention is our Co-Impact Sourcing® initiative.

As a self-proclaimed tree-hugger, overall plant lover, and someone who cares about the planet and the people living on it, this piece of the puzzle has become the most important piece for me.

In addition to supplying the highest quality essential oils dōTERRA® is committed to making a positive difference in the lives of farmers, harvesters, and distillers who contribute to dōTERRA's oil production.

With over 100 essential oils in its product line, dōTERRA® sources its oils from over 40 countries — more than half of which could be considered developing countries. To ensure that small-scale farmers and harvesters in disadvantaged areas are treated ethically, dōTERRA® has introduced an initiative called Co-Impact Sourcing®.

Co-Impact Sourcing® is an initiative that seeks to develop long-term, mutually beneficial supplier partnerships while creating sustainable jobs and providing reliable income in underdeveloped areas. dōTERRA® is committed to the ethical treatment of its suppliers by providing on-time payments at fair prices. Growers and harvesters are encouraged to form cooperative groups to share collective benefits and bargaining power while improving skills and capacity.

Additionally, the Healing Hands Foundation, dōTERRA®'s charitable organization, provides funding and resources to create community-based, social-impact projects to improve lives in the larger communities where oils are sourced. Past projects include building or sponsoring existing medical clinics, installing drinking water and irrigation systems, building schools, and providing other educational resources such as vocational training programs.

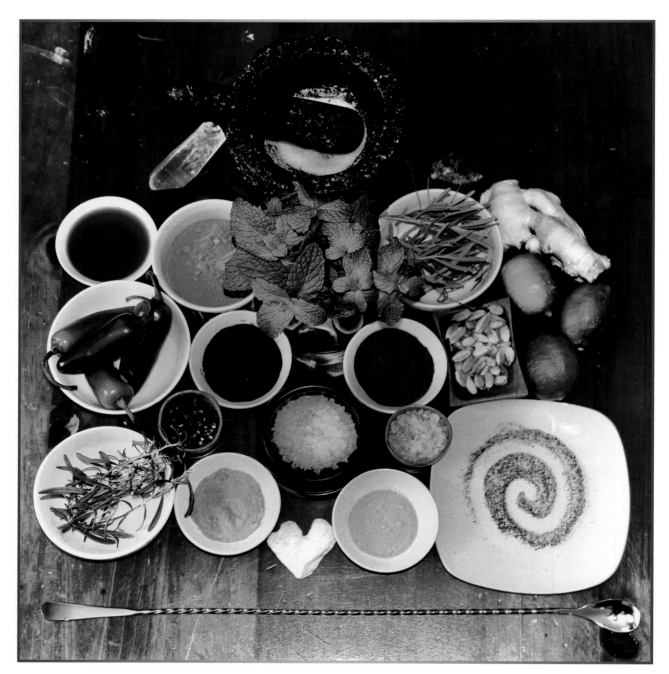

INGREDIENTS MATTER

Using quality ingredients is the foundation for creating a craft cocktail/mocktail elixir worthy of putting into our body temples. Therefore, choosing the highest quality spirits, juices, sugars, etc., is very important.

I have been told by some that when they follow my recipes, the end result still tastes different than what they experience with me. I always ask them what brand of alcohol they used, if they used fresh organic juice, or if they squeezed their own limes? They all respond the same - they used mass-produced spirits and/or did not choose other fresh quality ingredients. Please don't negate the importance of this - it will make all the difference in the end product.

THINK LIKE A PURIST

- **Choose artisan, small batch spirits.**
- **Stay away from mass-produced spirits from the larger companies, unless they are organic.**
- **Whenever possible, always choose organic for any ingredient.**
- **Whenever possible, choose to juice fresh fruits rather than buying the juice.**
- **If you can't juice fresh, choose organic brands.**
- **Never use white sugar to make simple syrup.**
- **Get familiar with honey, agave, maple syrup, raw cane, and coconut sugar.**
- **Stay away from traditional table salt.**
- **Get to know artisan salts: Himalayan salt, Fleur de Sel, etc.**
- **Only use dōTERRA® CPTG® essential oils.**
- **Tonic water can be a black hole ingredient. Choose a good one — I like Fever Tree.**
- **Read labels. You would be surprised at what they call food.**

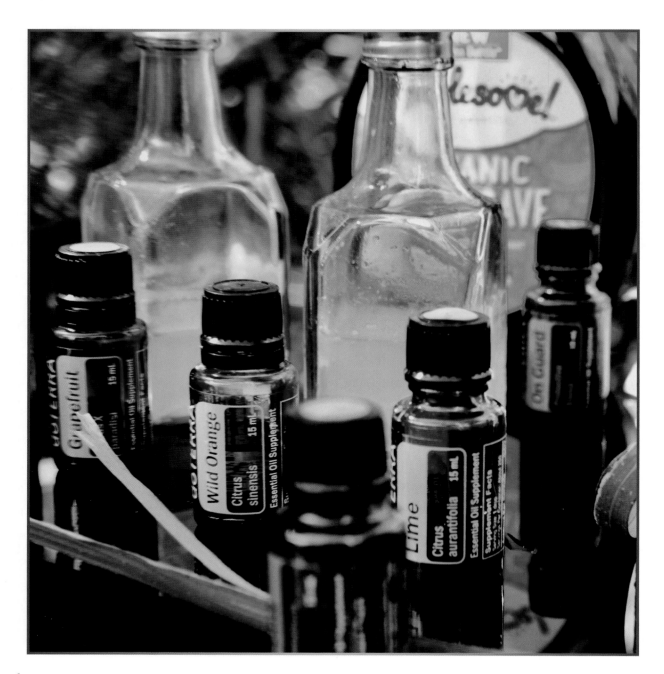

ROADMAP

In order for you to easily navigate the amazing recipes in this book with total ease, I have provided some definitions, tool suggestions, mixer recipes, instructions and suggestions to support your journey.

TRADITIONAL SIMPLE SYRUP

Add 1 cup of boiling water to 1 cup of sugar of your choice and mix until the sugar has completely dissolved. Let the mixture cool and then refrigerate in an airtight glass container. Keeps for up to 1 month.

ESSENTIAL OIL-INFUSED SIMPLE SYRUP

Use the simple syrup created in the above recipe and add 2-3 drops of your chosen dōTERRA® essential oil.

HOMEMADE LEMONADE

Warm 10 cups of spring water in a saucepan, and keep it just below simmering. Add 1 cup of raw honey. Stir until it dissolves, and then let the mixture cool. Add the juice of 8 lemons, stir thoroughly, and distribute into 16-ounce glass bottles. Cover tightly and store in the refrigerator for later use.

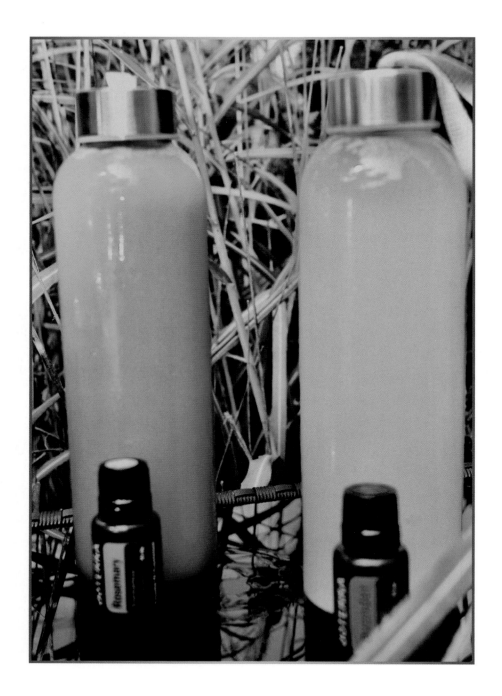

LAVENDER-INFUSED LEMONADE

Add 2-3 drops of dōTERRA® lavender essential oil to 16-ounce jars of homemade lemonade recipe. Cover tightly and store in the refrigerator for later use.

ROSEMARY-INFUSED PEACH NECTAR

Add 2-3 drops of dōTERRA® rosemary essential oil to a 16-ounce jar of peach nectar. Cover tightly and store in the refrigerator for later use.

YLANG YLANG INFUSED MANDARIN JUICE

Add 2 drops of dōTERRA® ylang ylang essential oil to a 16-ounce jar of mandarin juice. Cover tightly and store in the refrigerator for later use.

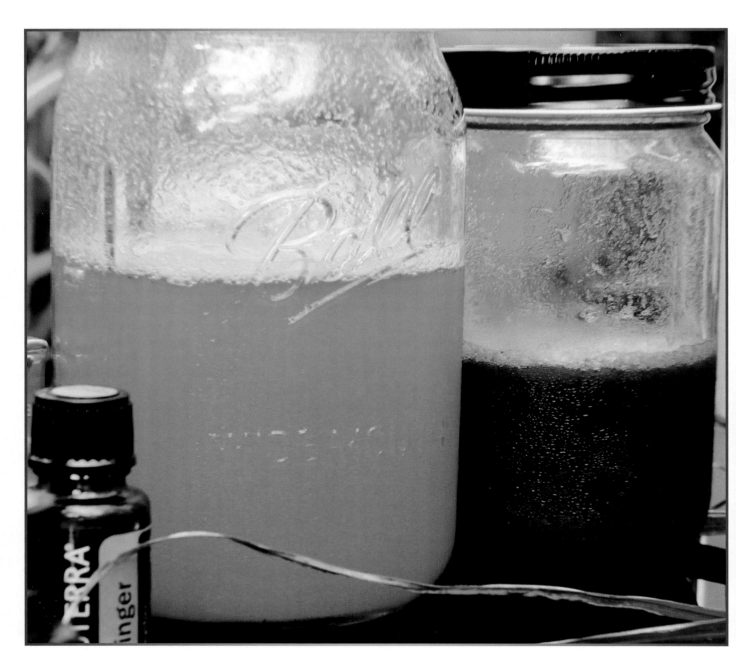

Cucumber Juice

In my experience, English cucumbers have the most flavor, but any kind will work. Peel and cut one cucumber. Place in Vitamix or blender. Add 2 cups of fresh spring water. Blend and place in a mason jar. Cover tightly and store in the refrigerator for later use.

Spinach Juice

Fill your blender or Vitamix to the top with organic spinach, add 2 cups of water, and blend until it's a liquid consistency. Place in a mason jar, cover tightly and store in the refrigerator for later use.

Bottle Suggestions

Mason jars work well for storing juice. I also like to save old kombucha bottles — they are usually 16 ounces and make the perfect mixing bottle. When making simple syrups, I often buy vinegar bottles or just use a mason jar or kombucha bottle. It's a good practice to label the bottles since you could be making several things at once. Knowing what's what will eliminate confusion at a later date.

Rose Water

Rose water can be found in most specialty grocery stores. If not, it can easily be ordered online.

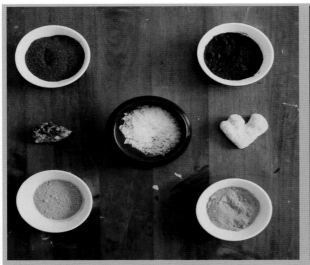
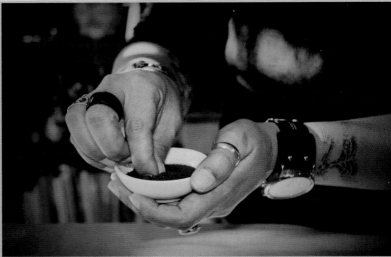
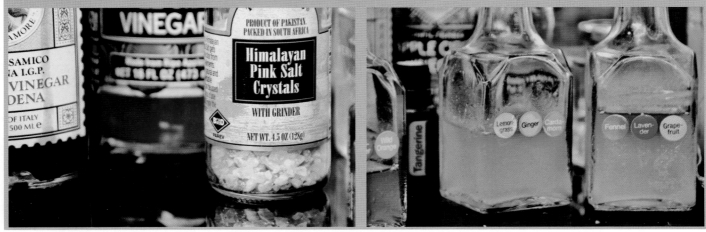

SALTS

A couple of my recipes call for Himalayan Salt and Fleur de Sel. Himalayan salt comes from the Himalayan mountains. It can be found in most grocery stores these days or can be ordered online. It's rich in minerals and considered by some to be very beneficial to the body. Fleur de Sel is called the "flower of salt" and is a very special finishing salt that can be found in most specialty grocery stores.

TOOTHPICK METHOD

Essential oils pack a lot of flavor. It's important to remember that a little goes a long way and that less is always more. When I suggest the toothpick method, I want you to get a clean wooden toothpick and stick the toothpick through the top of the essential oil bottle, slightly dipping the tip of the toothpick into the bottle. Do not immerse the toothpick, just dip the tip. Then, take the toothpick and swirl it into the mixture you are concocting. You will be surprised by how much flavor this method creates.

MIXOLOGIST TOOL KIT

One can always choose to wing it, but, just as using quality ingredients matters, having the right tools will truly create better results. Invest in a cocktail shaker, a strainer, a double-sided jigger (2 ounces and 1 ounce), and a bar spoon. I personally use a **Boston Shaker** and Hawthorn Strainer, but that's just my preference.

ADDITIONAL HELPERS

A zester, a lemon/lime press, a few 1-2-inch square ice cube trays and a nice selection of glassware all come in handy. These additional things make it easier to get the results you want and create a better presentation, resulting in a better experience.

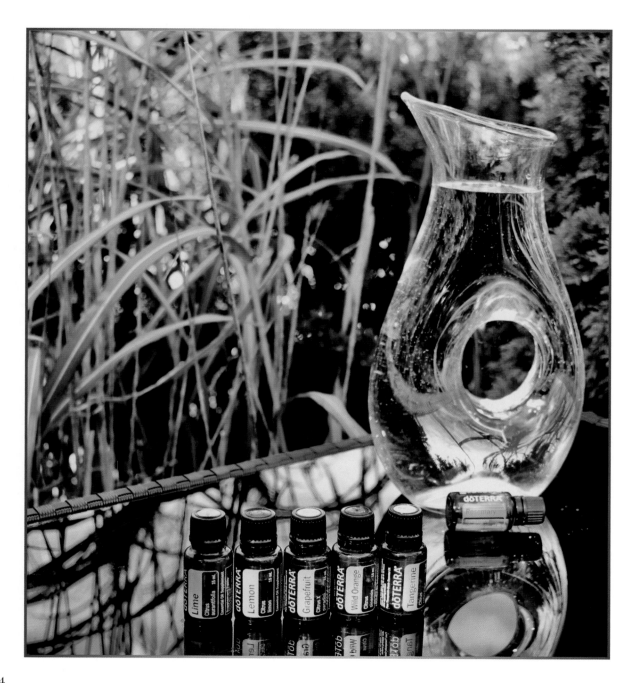

HYDRATION STATION

Water is the elixir of life. Without it, our cells dehydrate and aren't able to perform their duties within our body temples. It's important that we drink the right amount of water for our bodies each day. In addition, we need to drink additional water when we choose to imbibe a cocktail with alcohol.

When I have guests in our home and I have my Essential Mixologist hat on, I like to set up a little hydration station. I choose a beautiful glass pitcher and whatever dōTERRA® essential oil I feel like offering. I fill the pitcher with water and add 3-5 drops of the oil to the water. I always use glass since many of the citrus essential oils tend to leach BPA's from plastic and the whole point is to assist the body to rid itself of these toxic chemicals, not to add more.

My dōTERRA® essential oil suggestions for water are usually from the citrus family: Lemon, Lime, Grapefruit, Wild Orange, and Tangerine. I also use Rosemary since it further assists with detoxification, brings in a wonderful herbaceous element, and is stimulating to the mind. The combination of these oils always produces some nice flavor combinations, gives the body extra detox support and creates an uplifting aroma that's a consistent crowd pleaser.

Don't feel like you have to wait until you are serving cocktails to set up a hydration station in your home. We always have one set up, and we change the oils out according to our moods and the physical needs of the day. It's a fun way to change up your water routine!

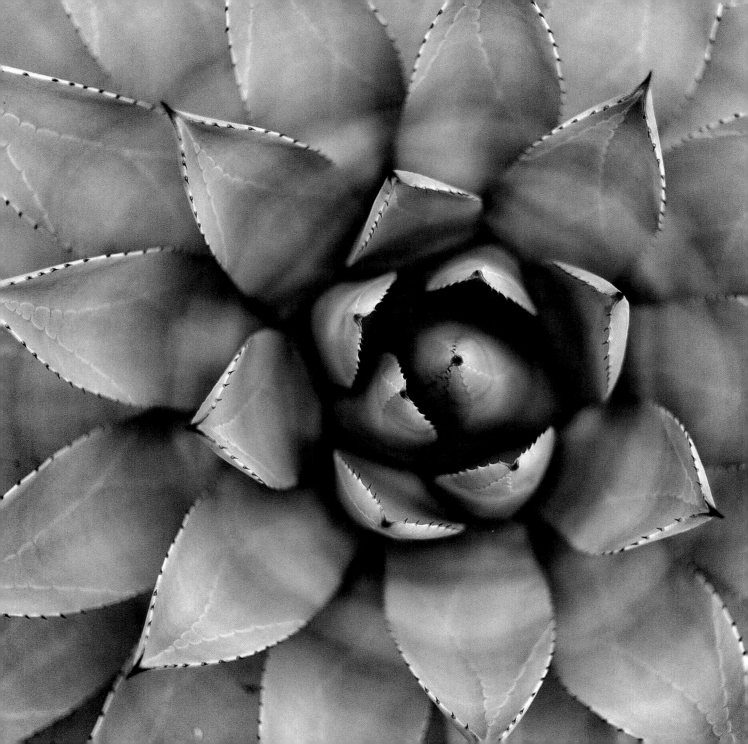

BLANCO ~ REPOSADO ~ ANEJO ~ MEZCAL

There's no other way to say it: I'm a tequila girl. When given the option, it's always my first choice. I love the complexities of this plant and I'm attracted to its energy and vibration. The agave plant and I seem to dance in harmony — it mixes well with my chemistry, and I love to play with the variety of expressions that come from it.

I won't provide this kind of detail for any other spirit, but since tequila has so many ways in which it expresses itself, I feel it's worth explaining further.

Here's a Tequila 101 breakdown for those interested in knowing the differences in how this plant expresses itself. There are more ways than those listed, but this a great start for anyone who is curious.

Blanco: tequila that's either aged for less than two months in stainless steel or neutral oak barrels or simply bottled or stored immediately after distillation. Some refer to it as silver tequila.

Reposado (rested): aged for a minimum of two months but for less than a year in oak barrels of any size.

Añejo (aged or vintage): aged for a minumum of one year but for less than three years in small oak barrels. This beauty is best left alone and served straight up like a good cognac, or over a few rocks and treated like a nice scotch.

Mezcal: distilled from any type of agave plant native to Mexico. The word mezcal means "oven-cooked agave." Mezcal has a very distinct smoky flavor that for many is an acquired taste.

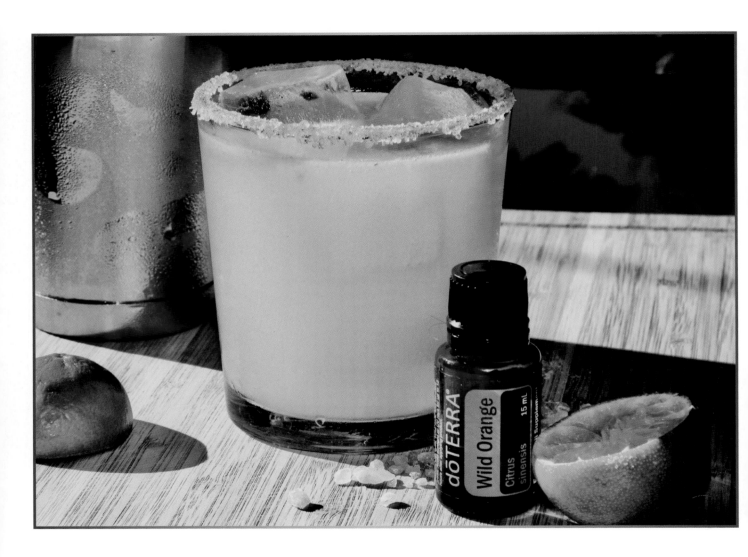

THE PURIST MARGARITA

2 ounces blanco tequila

2 fresh squeezed limes

1 squirt agave

2 drops dōTERRA® wild orange essential oil

garnish with Himalayan salt rim

Fill shaker with ice. Layer ingredients in shaker, shake well and serve in a rocks glass over ice.

WILD ORANGE ESSENTIAL OIL

Cold pressed from the peel, Wild Orange is one of dōTERRA®'s top-selling essential oils due to its energizing aroma and multiple health benefits. High in monoterpenes, Wild Orange possesses stimulating and purifying qualities, making it ideal to support a healthy immune system function. It can be taken daily to cleanse the body or used on surfaces as a natural cleaner. Diffusing Wild Orange will energize and uplift the mind and body while purifying the air.

PRIMARY BENEFITS

- energizing
- helps with anxiety
- mood enhancing

NOTES FROM JULEZ

Taking a sip from the perfect margarita is like getting on a magic carpet (at least what I would imagine a magic carpet to be like): a smooth, awe-inspiring journey of the senses. I tell people this goes beyond the "skinny margarita" since the wild orange brings in HUGE flavor with no additional calories. What I love about this cocktail/mocktail is its simplicity — it requires little effort for a big return. Everyone I have ever served this cocktail to (and there have been hundreds) says they feel energized and emotionally uplifted after just a few sips. Serve this with a little salsa, guacamole and some chips to dip and your guests will feel like they walked into the best cantina north of the border.

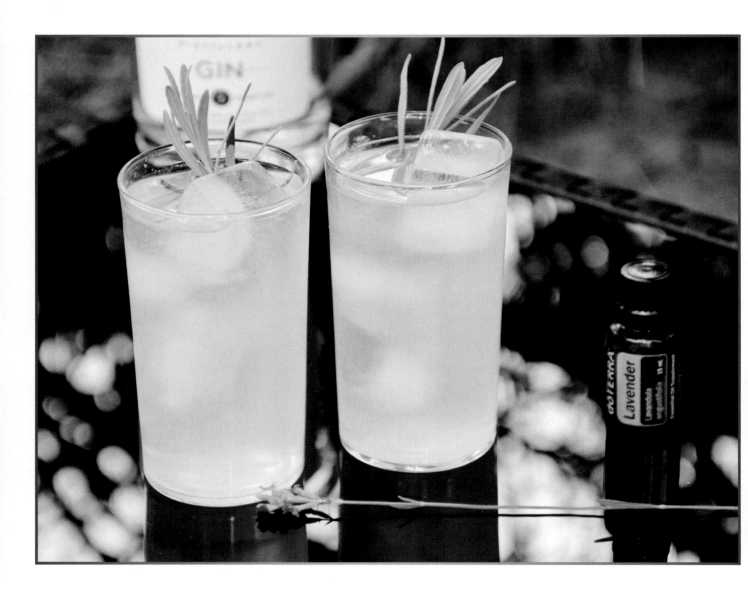

LAVENDER LEMONADE GIN FIZZ

2 ounces gin

4 ounces dōTERRA® lavender-infused lemonade

1 extra teaspoon of honey if you prefer a little sweeter

finish with fizzy water

garnish with a lavender sprig

Fill shaker with ice. Layer ingredients in shaker, stir well until it's very cold (gin is better stirred, not shaken). Serve over ice in a medium to tall glass. Fizzy water goes in last.

LAVENDER ESSENTIAL OIL

Lavender has been used and cherished for centuries for its unmistakable aroma and myriad benefits. In ancient times, the Egyptians and Romans used Lavender for bathing, relaxation, cooking, and as a perfume. Its calming and relaxing qualities, when taken internally, continue to be Lavender's most notable attributes. Applied topically, Lavender is frequently used to reduce the appearance of skin imperfections. Add to bath water to soak away stress or apply to the temples and the back of the neck. Add a few drops of Lavender to pillows, bedding, or bottoms of feet to relax and prepare for a restful night's sleep. Due to Lavender's versatile properties, it is considered the must-have oil to have on hand at all times.

PRIMARY BENEFITS

- helps with focus and concentration
- aids with stress and anxiety
- eases tension and relaxing

NOTES FROM JULEZ

Lavender is one of my favorite essential oils. I use it every day for many different reasons. I wanted to create a cocktail that highlights the beauty of this plant. Because gin is so incredibly botanical, it was the ideal spirit choice to alchemize with the perfection that is lavender. What I love about this cocktail/mocktail is how it truly embodies the energy of unwinding. It's literally magic in a glass and is wonderful at the end of a hectic day. The lavender is nurturing to the body and mind: it really puts you on another frequency. It's the perfect drink to serve with appetizers: cheeses, nuts, etc. The lavender is a culinary compliment to just about anything one would snack on over cocktails.

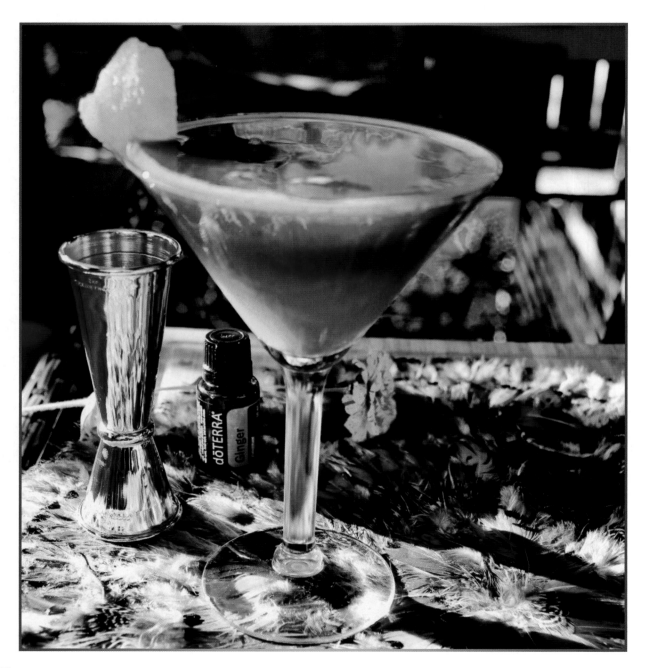

AFRICAN SUNSET

2 ounces reposado tequila

4 ounces cherry juice

1/2 fresh squeezed lime

1/2 teaspoon balsamic vinegar

1 squirt agave

1 drop dōTERRA® ginger essential oil

a dollop of mango nectar floated on top

garnish with a slice of candied ginger on rim

Fill shaker with ice. Layer ingredients in shaker, shake well and serve very cold, straight up in a martini glass. Pour mango nectar last slowly over the back of a spoon.

GINGER ESSENTIAL OIL

Newly sourced from Madagascar, dōTERRA® Ginger essential oil is derived from the fresh rhizome of the ginger plant—the subterranean stalk of a plant that shoots out the root system. A featured ingredient in many Asian dishes, Ginger has a hot, fragrant flavor when used as a kitchen spice. In Western tradition, Ginger is most often used in sweets—gingerbread and ginger snaps being two examples. Internal use of Ginger is best known as a digestive aid and for helping to ease occasional indigestion and nausea. Ginger essential oil can also be applied topically or inhaled for a soothing aroma.

PRIMARY BENEFITS

- supports healthy digestion
- memory support
- anti-inflammatory

NOTES FROM JULEZ

What I love about this cocktail/mocktail is its beauty. It makes a stunning presentation when the mango nectar is floated correctly. I suggest turning a spoon backwards because it slows the pour. The trick is to get the nectar to trickle into the glass so that it doesn't mix with the rest of the drink and gives it a dramatic look, just like an African sunset. I chose the name African Sunset in honor of the dōTERRA® ginger essential oil that is sourced from Madagascar, and because the look of this drink really does resemble the most beautiful African sunset. Keep in mind that this cocktail makes a wonderful aperitif since the ginger can get the digestive juices flowing and stimulate an appetite. (An aperitif is a drink had before a meal to stimulate the appetite.) It also makes a wonderful after-dinner cocktail since the ginger can act as a "digestivo" and aid in the digestion of the meal.

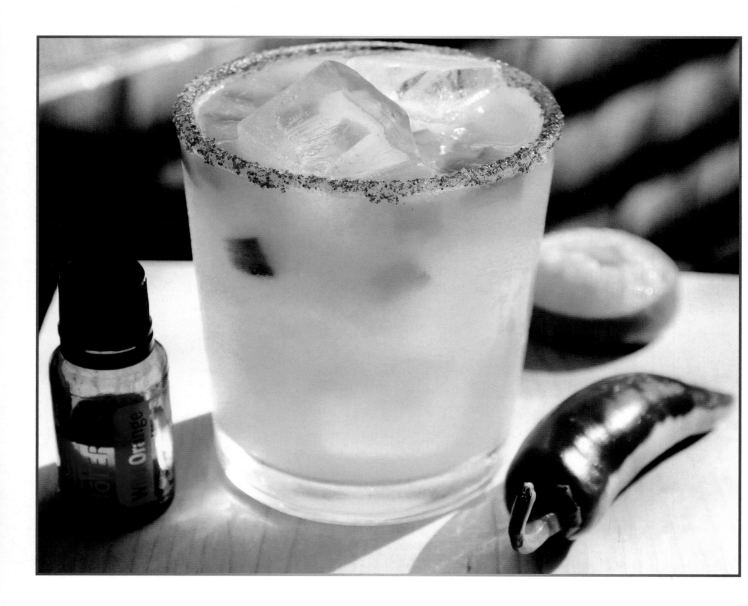

THE REBEL PURIST

2 ounces blanco tequila

3 ounces fresh cucumber juice

1/2 fresh squeezed lime

1/2 teaspoon fresh jalapeño juice

1 squirt agave

2 drops dōTERRA® wild orange essential oil

garnish with Himalayan/ancho chili powder salt rim and diced cucumber chunks

Fill shaker with ice. Layer ingredients in shaker, shake well and serve in a rocks glass over ice.

WILD ORANGE ESSENTIAL OIL

Cold pressed from the peel, Wild Orange is one of dōTERRA®'s top-selling essential oils due to its energizing aroma and multiple health benefits. High in monoterpenes, Wild Orange possesses stimulating and purifying qualities, making it ideal to support healthy immune system function. It can be taken daily to cleanse the body or used on surfaces as a natural cleaner. Diffusing Wild Orange will energize and uplift the mind and body while purifying the air.

PRIMARY BENEFITS

- energizing
- helps with anxiety
- mood enhancing

NOTES FROM JULEZ

What I love about this cocktail/mocktail is its ability to catapult anyone into the category of mixologist. If there's any intimidation around making the cucumber juice — get over it! It's super easy and well worth the small amount of effort. Remember, make extra and save it in a mason jar in the refrigerator for other cocktails. One of my tricks for getting juice from the jalapeño is cutting it into small chunks and putting them into my lime press. You can also cut the jalapeño into pieces, place into the Vitamix or blender and add a small amount of water. Blend, and then strain and store in a small jar. A little of this goes a long way! A tip for salting the rim of the glass is to mix the Himalayan salt and ancho chili powder on a plate, rub a lime or even a little agave syrup over the rim of the glass, and then rub the glass into the salt and chili powder mixture.

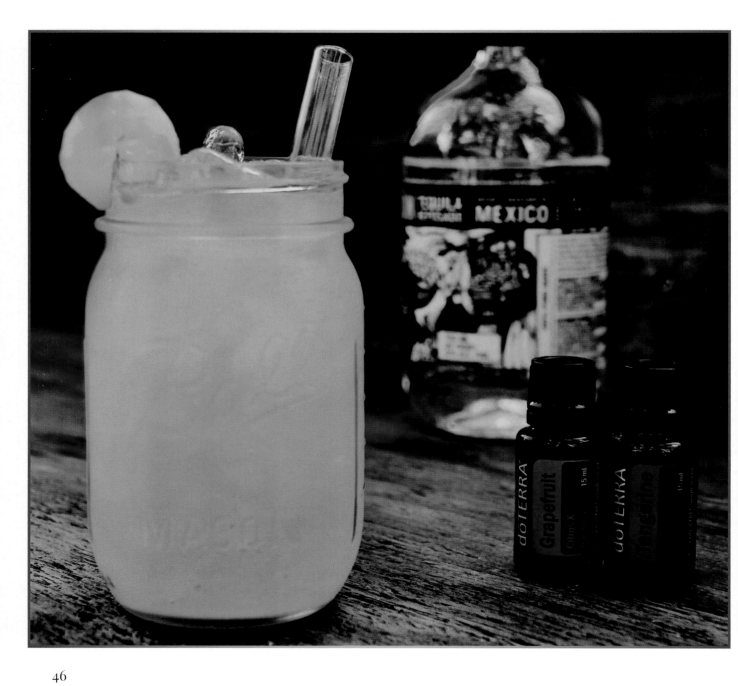

A VERY REFRESHING COCKTAIL

2 ounces blanco tequila

3 ounces cucumber juice

1/2 fresh squeezed lime

1/4 teaspoon rose water

1 squirt agave

2 drops dōTERRA® grapefruit essential oil

2 drops dōTERRA® tangerine essential oil

garnish with a cucumber slice

Fill shaker with ice. Layer ingredients in shaker, shake well and serve in a mason jar or rocks glass over ice.

GRAPEFRUIT ESSENTIAL OIL

Referred to as a "forbidden fruit" and one of the "Seven Wonders of Barbados," Grapefruit was first documented in 1750 by Welshman Rev. Griffith Hughes. Known for its energizing and invigorating aroma, Grapefruit helps uplift mood. Grapefruit is also renowned for its cleansing and purifying properties and is frequently used in skin care for its ability to promote the appearance of clear, healthy-looking skin.

PRIMARY BENEFITS

- supports adrenal recovery
- reduces sugar cravings
- supports healthy metabolism

TANGERINE ESSENTIAL OIL

Tangerine has a long history of use in Chinese culture and herbal health practices. Tangerine has a sweet, tangy aroma, similar to other citrus oils, that is uplifting. Tangerine is known for its cleansing properties, and for supporting a healthy immune and respiratory system. Tangerine essential oil can be used to help soothe anxious feelings and manage stress.

PRIMARY BENEFITS

- supports healthy digestion and metabolism
- cleansing and purifying
- supports a healthy immune system

NOTES FROM JULEZ

What I love about this cocktail/mocktail is everything. If you could actually drink a day at the spa, this is what it would taste like. I call it "A Very Refreshing Cocktail" because almost everyone I serve it to takes a sip and says, "this is such a refreshing cocktail". Cucumber water is cooling, hydrating and a wonderful thirst quencher. This drink also makes a superb mocktail: it's one of my favorites to sip on without alcohol. Consider making it by the pitcher for those summer outdoor parties — your guests will be very impressed.

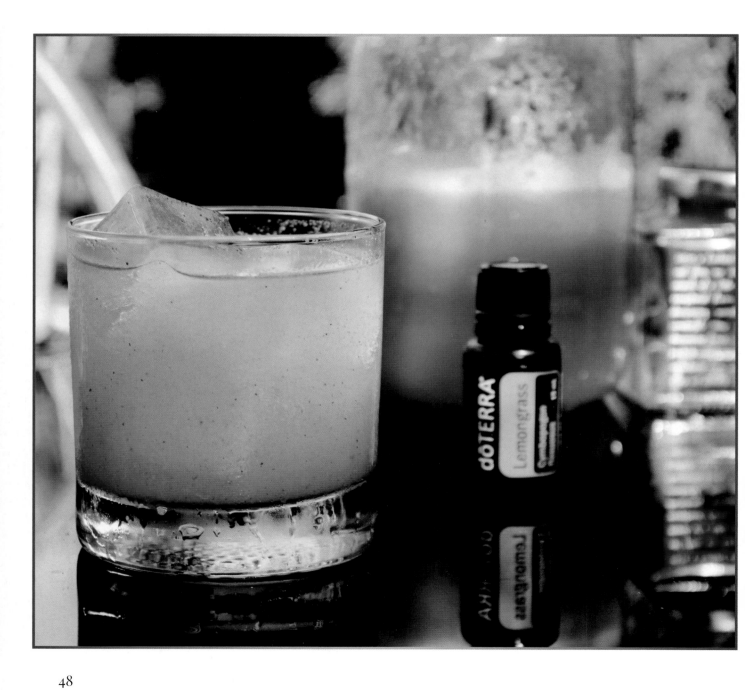

GRASSY KNOLL

1 1/2 ounces reposado tequila

2 ounces sake

2 ounces cucumber juice

1/2 fresh squeezed lime

1 tablespoon lemongrass simple syrup

1 pinch chipotle powder

Fill shaker with ice. Layer ingredients in shaker, shake well and serve in a rocks glass over ice, or straight up in a martini or coupe glass — your choice.

LEMONGRASS ESSENTIAL OIL

A tall, perennial plant, Lemongrass has a subtle citrus flavor and is used in Asian cuisine in soups, teas, and curries as well as with fish, poultry, beef, and seafood. In addition to its unique flavor, Lemongrass essential oil promotes healthy digestion and acts as an overall tonic to the body's systems when ingested. It's also purifying and toning to the skin, and is frequently used in skin care products for these benefits. Lemongrass is an ideal oil to use in massage therapy. Lemongrass has a pungent, herbaceous aroma that can heighten awareness and promote a positive outlook.

PRIMARY BENEFITS

- promotes a healthy outlook
- overall tonic for the body
- helps with circulation and digestion

NOTES FROM JULEZ

I have always found lemongrass to be an essential oil that makes my heart happy. What I love about this cocktail/mocktail is that it reminds me of my plant medicine roots at Herbalicious. We used to brew a lemongrass tea and we called it "Happy Tea". There's something about the herbaceous notes along with the citrus that puts a smile on my face every time. This cocktail stands alone, but because of the Asian flavor profile of the lemongrass and the sake, I love to serve it with sushi. People think I named this drink after the famous grassy knoll from the Kennedy shooting. I didn't. I love finding a grassy knoll the lay on and connect with the earth. It's my happy place and that's what the drink is named after, my happy place.

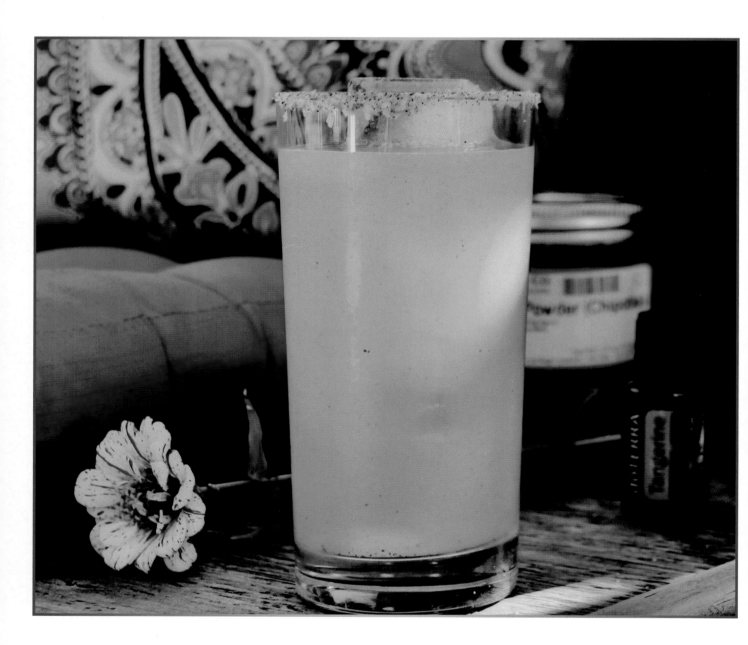

DULCE PICANTE

2 ounces reposado tequila

3 ounces passion fruit juice

1/2 fresh squeezed lime

1 squirt agave

2 drops dōTERRA® tangerine oil

pinch of spicy chipotle powder

garnish with chipotle/Himalayan salt rim

Fill shaker with ice. Layer ingredients in shaker, shake well and serve in a medium tall glass over ice.

TANGERINE ESSENTIAL OIL

Tangerine has a long history of use in Chinese culture and herbal health practices. The essential oil supports healthy digestion and metabolism. Tangerine has a sweet, tangy aroma, similar to other citrus oils, that is uplifting. Tangerine is known for its cleansing properties, and for supporting a healthy immune and respiratory system. Tangerine essential oil can be used to help soothe anxious feelings and manage stress. A popular and flavorful addition to desserts and drinks—from water to fruit smoothies—Tangerine can be used in any recipe calling for citrus fruits.

PRIMARY BENEFITS

- cleansing and purifying
- supports a healthy immune system
- supports healthy digestion and metabolism

NOTES FROM JULEZ

Passion fruit is one of my favorite flavors on the planet and this cocktail was born from my passion for these very specific flavors. What I love about this cocktail/mocktail is its unique floral note and how that mixes with the smoky/spicy quality of the chipotle. I just love the way these sweet and spicy flavors come together with the semi-aged quality of reposado tequila. Don't be shy about putting a healthy pinch of chipotle into the drink. It definitely adds to the flavor profile and the red flecks look beautiful floating in the glass.

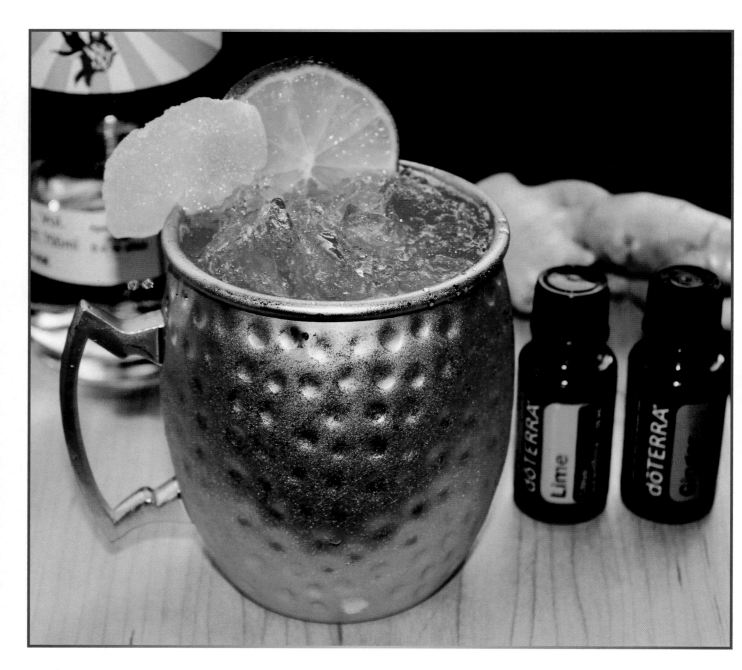

MEZCAL MULE

2 ounces mezcal

3 ounces lemonade

1/2 teaspoon apple cider vinegar

1 squirt agave nectar

1 drop dōTERRA® ginger essential oil

1 drop dōTERRA® lime essential oil

finish with fizzy water

garnish with a slice of candied ginger and a lime wheel

Fill shaker with ice. Layer ingredients in shaker, shake well and serve in a copper mug. Fizzy water goes in last.

GINGER ESSENTIAL OIL

Internal use of Ginger is best known as a digestive aid and for helping to ease occasional indigestion and nausea. Ginger essential oil can also be applied topically or inhaled for a soothing aroma.

PRIMARY BENEFITS

- supports healthy digestion
- memory support
- anti-inflammatory

LIME ESSENTIAL OIL

Cold-pressed from the peel of fresh limes, dōTERRA® Lime essential oil is refreshing and energizing in both aroma and taste. Due to its high limonene content, Lime provides internal cleansing benefits and can be diffused to help purify the air. It's also an effective and natural surface cleaner. Lime is known for its ability to uplift, balance, and energize.

PRIMARY BENEFITS

- supports healthy immune function
- used as an internal cleanser
- promotes emotional balance and well-being

NOTES FROM JULEZ

What I love about this cocktail/mocktail is that it represents the freedom to explore flavors. The foundation of a "mule" can take a mixologist in so many unique directions. Personally, I'm in love with the smoky flavor profile of mezcal, and I think it works well as a mule spirit. The ginger and lime essential oil support both digestion and the immune system, and with the addition of apple cider vinegar, it's the perfect elixir for any season. The copper mug isn't mandatory, but it certainly makes for a nice presentation.

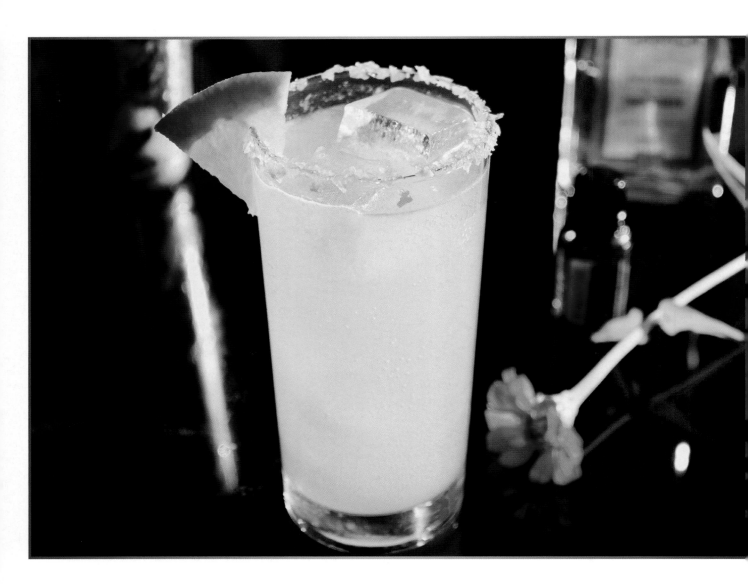

SMOKEY PALOMA

2 ounces mezcal

1 fresh squeezed lime

1 squirt agave

3 drops dōTERRA® grapefruit essential oil

5 ounces fizzy water

Fleur de Sel rim

Fill shaker with ice. Layer ingredients in shaker, shake well and serve over ice in a medium to tall glass. Fizzy water goes in last.

GRAPEFRUIT ESSENTIAL OIL

Referred to as a "forbidden fruit" and one of the "Seven Wonders of Barbados," Grapefruit was first documented in 1750 by Welshman Rev. Griffith Hughes. The name "grapefruit" is attributed to the fruits growing in clusters which resemble those of grapes. Known for its energizing and invigorating aroma, Grapefruit helps uplift mood. Grapefruit is also renowned for its cleansing and purifying properties and is frequently used in skin care for its ability to promote the appearance of clear, healthy-looking skin. Grapefruit can also support a healthy metabolism.

PRIMARY BENEFITS

- supports adrenal recovery
- reduces sugar cravings
- supports a healthy metabolism

NOTES FROM JULEZ

Palomas are a very traditional Mexican cocktail and are usually made with Jarritos, a grapefruit flavored soda loaded with white sugar. What I love about this cocktail/mocktail is that it's another expression of a purist mindset. The smoky flavor of the mezcal alchemizes with the dōTERRA® grapefruit essential oil, creating an opera on the palate. With the addition of the grapefruit essential oil, this cocktail is a wonderful support to our metabolisms. Anyone who is counting calories and watching their weight will really appreciate this drink. It's also a great daytime or pre-dinner drink to get the metabolic juices flowing. If you don't enjoy the flavor profile of mezcal, feel free to substitute with blanco or reposado tequila instead. In fact, it's actually what most traditional Palaomas use. The substitution of the mezcal is my happy rendition. Arribas!

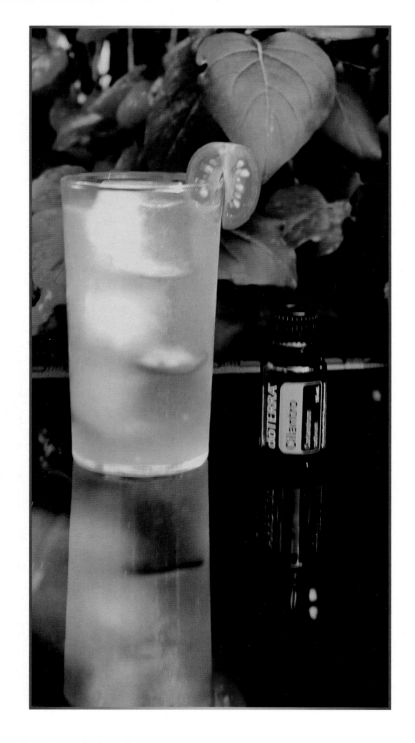

ODE TO THE DRUNKEN BOTANIST

2 ounces gin

1 tablespoon cucumber juice

3 thin slices jalapeño

toothpick method of dōTERRA® cilantro essential oil

finish with Fever-Tree tonic

garnish with a ripe cherry tomato

Fill shaker with ice. Layer ingredients in shaker. Dip toothpick top into the cilantro essential oil and mix into gin, stir well until very cold (gin is better stirred, not shaken). Layer the jalapeño slices between the cubes of ice in a medium to tall glass. Tonic water goes in last.

CILANTRO ESSENTIAL OIL

The culinary uses and additional benefits of Cilantro have been documented for centuries. Internal use of Cilantro promotes healthy digestion and supports healthy immune and nervous system functions. Applied topically, Cilantro is very soothing and cooling to the skin and it adds a fresh, herbal aroma to any essential oil blend when diffused.

PRIMARY BENEFITS

- supports healthy digestion
- powerful cleanser
- powerful detoxifier

NOTES FROM JULEZ

This cocktail is in honor of one of my mixology heroes, Amy Stewart, who wrote an amazing book called The Drunken Botanist. Amy is a genius when it comes to plants and the botanical world. If you are interested in taking a deeper dive, I highly recommend getting a copy of her book. I have to give her all of the credit here: I modified with dōTERRA® cilantro essential oil because that's what I do. I also juiced my cucumber as opposed to muddling, but this recipe comes from her artistic wellspring — hence the name "Ode to the Drunken Botanist". What I love about this cocktail/mocktail is that it's perfect. There are a couple of things I will say about this drink: use the toothpick method for the Cilantro essential oil. This stuff is really strong, and even one small drop would overpower the entire drink...trust me. Slice the jalapeño and layer one slice on the bottom of the glass, and the next one on top of the next cube and another on top of the next cube. Three slices seem to be sufficient. If you want extra spice, you can add another and also leave the seeds in. If you want less spice, remove the seeds, since that's where most of the heat lives in hot peppers. Enjoy this drink anytime — I love it in the afternoon with snacks. It beckons to be sipped in a garden while listening to Pink Martini, at least for me.

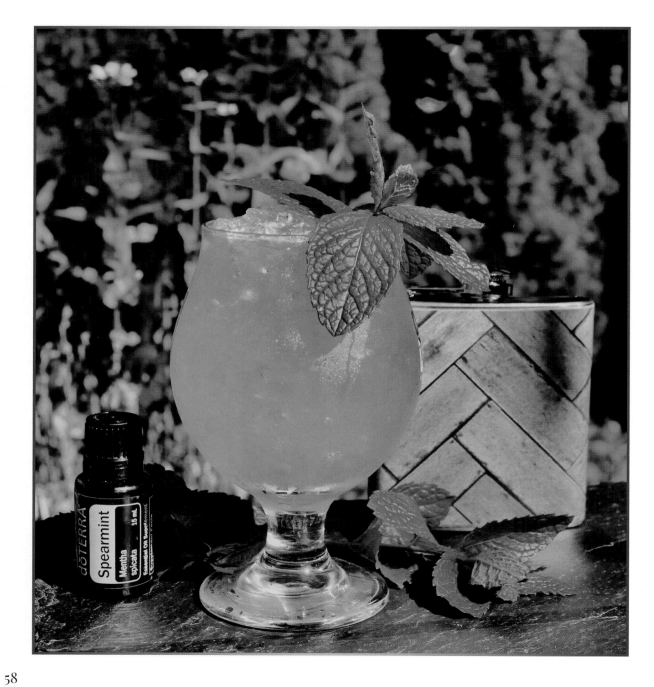

JULEZ JULEP

2 ounces bourbon

2 ounces cucumber juice

1/2 fresh squeezed lime

1 tablespoon maple syrup

1 drop dōTERRA® spearmint essential oil

finish with fizzy water

garnish with a sprig of mint

Fill shaker with ice. Layer ingredients in shaker, stir well and serve over crushed ice in glass of choice. I prefer a brandy snifter.

SPEARMINT ESSENTIAL OIL

Spearmint is a perennial plant that grows 11–40 inches tall and flourishes in temperate climates. It is widely used in gums, candies, and dental products for its minty taste, and to promote fresh breath. Spearmint has been used for centuries for its digestive benefits. Its sweet, refreshing aroma is cleansing and uplifting, making it ideal to evoke a sense of focus and positive mood. Spearmint is very different from Peppermint, making it a milder option to use on children and those with sensitive skin. In cooking, Spearmint is frequently used in salads, drinks, and desserts, but it can also be used in homemade salad dressings and to marinate meats.

PRIMARY BENEFITS

- reduces occasional stomach upset
- promotes a sense of focus and uplifts mood
- cleanses the mouth and promotes fresh breath

NOTES FROM JULEZ

What I love about this cocktail/mocktail is its story. The first time I had a mint julep was when we were visiting my wife's family in Kentucky. It sounds cliché, but it's true. We sat outside and sipped these very strong concoctions of bourbon and artificial-tasting mint. I thought, there has to be a better way. It wasn't my in-laws' fault: by mint julep standards, that cocktail was probably right up there with the best of them. However, I'm a purist, so I'm always looking for ways to find the flavor in its purest form. dōTERRA's® spearmint essential oil is divine and as pure as it gets. I have modified the traditional recipe a little — after all, it is a Julez Julep — but I feel the additions work nicely. I'm not sure if the Julez Julep would be accepted at the Kentucky Derby, but I would love to have the opportunity.

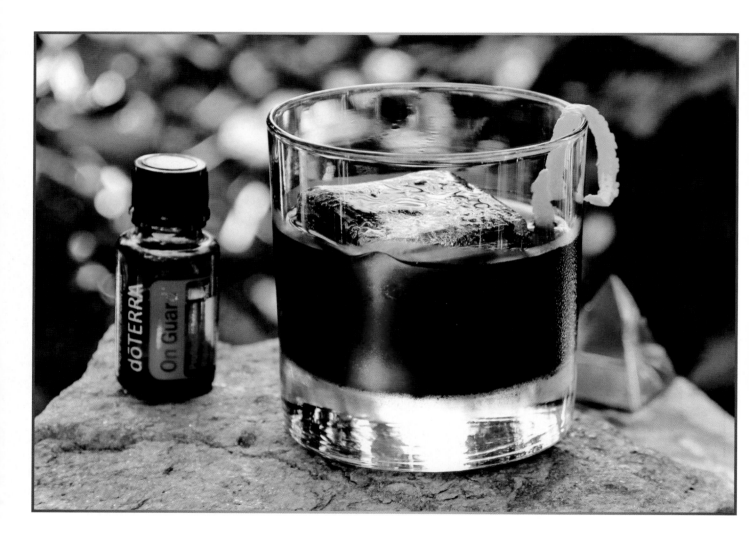

NEW AGE OLD FASHIONED

2 ounces whiskey or rye

3 ounces cherry juice

1/2 fresh squeezed lemon

1 drop dōTERRA® On Guard® Blend

garnish with an orange rind or a real cherry

1 teaspoon maple syrup (for a sweeter preference)

Fill shaker with ice. Layer ingredients in shaker, stir well and serve over ice (I like to use one 2.5-inch square cube) in a rocks glass.

ON GUARD® ESSENTIAL OIL BLEND

dōTERRA® On Guard®, a proprietary essential oil blend, provides a natural and effective alternative for immune support when used internally. As one of dōTERRA®'s best-selling blends, dōTERRA® On Guard® protects against environmental and seasonal threats with essential oils known for their positive effects on the immune system when ingested. dōTERRA® On Guard® can be taken internally on a daily basis to maintain healthy immune function and support healthy cardiovascular function. It can also be used on surfaces throughout the home as a non-toxic cleaner. When diffused, dōTERRA® On Guard® helps purify the air and can be very energizing and uplifting.

NOTES FROM JULEZ

The brown (whiskey) has totally made its way back into the modern cocktail movement. Every time I sip a whiskey-based cocktail, it gives me the feeling of traversing back in time. I feel the energy of a speak-easy in each sip, and when I come to my senses, I'm always amazed I'm not somewhere in the 1920's and am instead sitting in a hip cocktail bar in the new millennium — hence the name "New Age Old Fashioned". What I love about this cocktail/mocktail is the flavor profile that the dōTERRA® On Guard® Blend brings and the immune enhancing properties it naturally has. This drink truly is an immune supporting elixir. It makes a wonderful nightcap and gives your body a little extra support before you turn in for your evening slumber. Yeah, I said slumber. I think it's something they would have said in the 1920's.

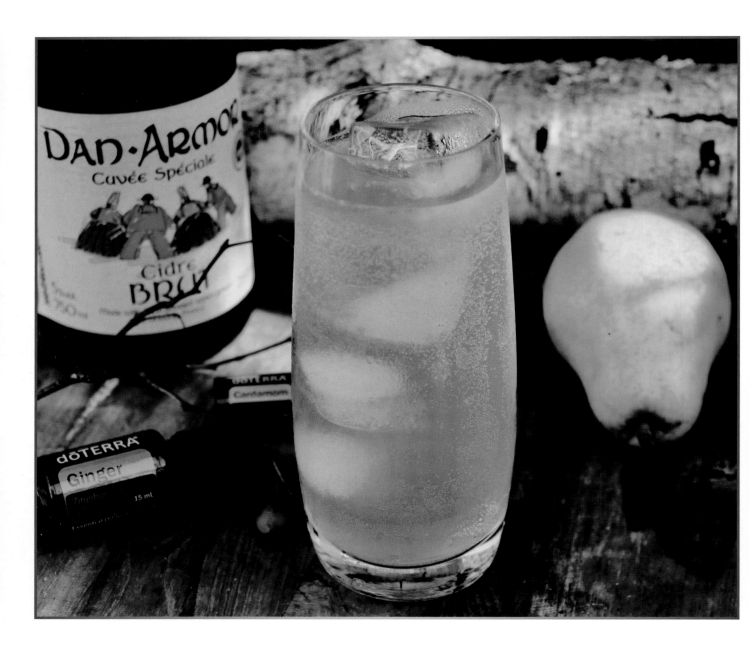

SPICED FALL FIZZ

2 ounces whiskey or rye

1 ounce Poire Williams pear brandy

1 drop dōTERRA® ginger essential oil

1 drop dōTERRA® cardamom essential oil

finish with hard apple cider

Fill shaker with ice. Layer ingredients in shaker, stir well and serve over ice in a tall glass. Hard apple cider goes in last.

GINGER ESSENTIAL OIL

Ginger is known for helping to ease indigestion and nausea. Ginger essential oil can also be applied topically or inhaled for a soothing aroma.

PRIMARY BENEFITS

- supports healthy digestion
- memory support
- anti-inflammatory

CARDAMOM ESSENTIAL OIL

A close relative to Ginger, Cardamom is known as an expensive cooking spice and for being beneficial to the digestive system in a variety of ways. Cardamom is commonly used internally to help soothe occasional stomach discomfort. Its distinct scent can promote a positive mood. Ingested Cardamom also has profound effects on the respiratory system due to its high 1,8-cineole content, which promotes clear breathing and respiratory health. Native to Southeast Asia, Cardamom is added to traditional Indian sweets and teas for its cool, minty aroma and flavor. dōTERRA® Cardamom essential oil is extracted from Cardamom seeds grown in Guatemala, using our strict CPTG® testing standards.

PRIMARY BENEFITS

- helps maintain gastrointestinal health
- promotes clear breathing
- promotes overall respiratory health

NOTES FROM JULEZ

I love the fall, especially the beautiful colors of the foliage and the crisp clean air that it brings to New England. It beckons for a really delicious cocktail filled with the fruits of autumn: freshly picked apples and pears. What I love about this cocktail/mocktail is how it tastes like fall in a glass. It's perfect for any occasion where the moment strikes you. Please feel free to replace the hard cider with non-alcoholic cider. It makes for a lovely pre-Thanksgiving dinner drink. The ginger and cardamom create a good setup for some nice assistance in the digestion department, making seconds a no-brainer, or even helping you save room for a slice of mom's pumpkin pie.

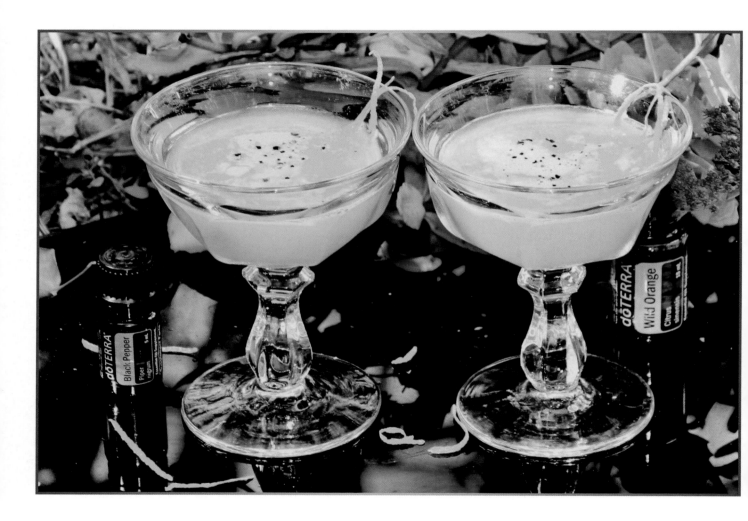

MARMALADE ZING

2 ounces dark rum
3 ounces fresh squeezed orange juice
1 teaspoon of honey
1 teaspoon apple cider vinegar
1 drop dōTERRA® black pepper essential oil
2 drops dōTERRA® wild orange essential oil
garnish with orange zest & black pepper pinch

Fill shaker with ice. Layer ingredients in shaker, shake well and serve cold in a coupe glass.

BLACK PEPPER ESSENTIAL OIL

Black Pepper is best known as a common cooking spice that enhances the flavor of foods, but its internal and topical benefits are equally noteworthy. This essential oil is high in monoterpenes and sesquiterpenes, known for their antioxidant activity and ability to help ward off environmental and seasonal threats. Black Pepper should be used with caution when applied topically due to its strong warming sensation. It can also help with the digestion of foods, making it an ideal oil to cook with and enjoy both for its flavor and internal benefits.

PRIMARY BENEFITS

• provides antioxidant support
• supports healthy circulation and digestion
• soothes anxious feelings

WILD ORANGE ESSENTIAL OIL

Cold pressed from the peel, Wild Orange is one of dōTERRA®'s top-selling essential oils due to its energizing aroma and multiple health benefits. High in monoterpenes, Wild Orange possesses stimulating and purifying qualities, making it ideal to support a healthy immune system function. It can be taken daily to cleanse the body or used on surfaces as a natural cleaner. Diffusing Wild Orange will energize and uplift the mind and body while purifying the air.

PRIMARY BENEFITS

• supports healthy digestion and metabolism
• cleansing and purifying
• supports a healthy immune system

NOTES FROM JULEZ

Here we have a cacophony of flavors that work nicely together. The black pepper essential oil adds a little zing that lands on the palate in a fun and playful way. What I love about this cocktail / mocktail is it truly tastes like marmalade in your mouth. Just imagine how delicious it would be if you could spread it on toast! In fact, if you used whole oranges instead of juice and threw all of the ingredie-nts into a pan with some coconut oil and reduced it down, you might just have something. I may try this — to be continued...

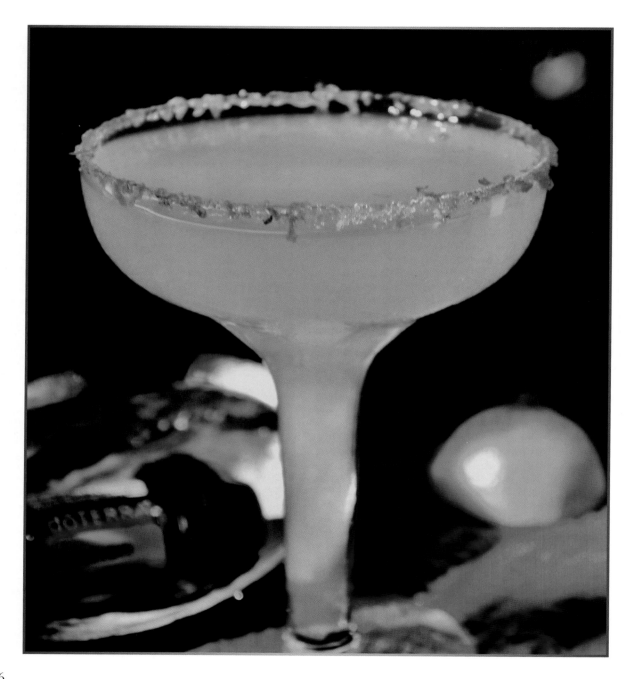

LEMON SQUIZZY

2 ounces vodka

4 ounces lemonade

1 squirt agave

2 drops dōTERRA® lemon essential oil

garnish rim with raw sugar & lemon zest

Fill shaker with ice. Layer ingredients in shaker, shake well and serve cold straight-up in a martini glass or a coupe glass.

LEMON ESSENTIAL OIL

The top-selling dōTERRA® essential oil, Lemon has multiple benefits and uses. Lemon is a powerful cleansing agent that purifies the air and surfaces and can be used as a non-toxic cleaner throughout the home. When added to water, Lemon provides a refreshing and healthy boost throughout the day. Lemon is frequently added to food to enhance the flavor of desserts and main dishes. Taken internally, Lemon provides cleansing and digestive benefits and supports healthy respiratory function. When diffused, Lemon is very uplifting and energizing and has been shown to help improve mood.

PRIMARY BENEFITS

- cleanses the body and aids in digestion
- supports healthy respiratory function
- promotes a positive mood

NOTES FROM JULEZ

Even though this cocktail reads nothing like a Cosmo, it feels like my offering as the successor of this now down-in-the-doldrums drink that seems to have gone out of style with the last episode of "Sex and the City" (which by the way I absolutely loved and watched all the time). I have a group of girlfriends who have been in my life since early childhood. We all have nicknames for one another (I won't share what mine was), and one of them is called Squiz. Squiz and I lived together in our twenties and drank our fair share of Cosmos together. I have a saying: "Easy breezy lemon Squizzy". I created this cocktail with her energy in mind. What I love about this cocktail/mocktail is that it's easy to make, has a sweet side and goes down smooth — and the double dose of lemon will brighten anyone's day. The Lemon essential oil also provides some detoxification support in case you forget that you're not Carrie Bradshaw and have more than just one of these. Cheers to old friends!

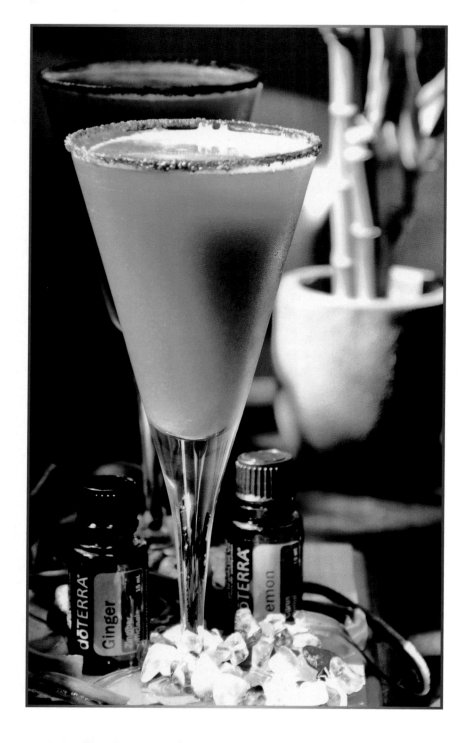

HEALTHY BUZZ

2 ounces blanco tequila or vodka

4 ounces fresh spinach juice

1 tablespoon honey

1 drop dōTERRA® ginger essential oil

2 drops dōTERRA® lemon essential oil

pinch of cayenne pepper powder

garish with spirulina and coconut sugar rim

Fill shaker with ice. Layer ingredients in shaker, shake well and serve very cold straight-up in a martini glass.

GINGER ESSENTIAL OIL

Ginger is known for helping to ease indigestion and nausea. Ginger essential oil can also be applied topically or inhaled for a soothing aroma.

PRIMARY BENEFITS

- supports healthy digestion
- memory support
- anti-inflammatory

LEMON ESSENTIAL OIL

Lemon is a powerful cleansing agent that purifies the air and surfaces. When added to water, Lemon provides a refreshing and healthy boost throughout the day. Taken internally, Lemon provides cleansing and digestive benefits and supports healthy respiratory function.

PRIMARY BENEFITS

- cleanses the body and aids in digestion
- supports healthy respiratory function
- promotes a positive mood

NOTES FROM JULEZ

What I love about this cocktail/mocktail is that it embodies the essence of my entire approach. It very easily makes a wonderful mocktail or healthy elixir. Everything about this drink screams healthy since it's such a huge support to the immune system and the digestive system — and with the fresh spinach juice, it's an amazing contribution to the whole body. This drink truly packs a nice energy boost. I would advise anyone who is feeling run-down to quadruple the recipe. Make a pitcher (minus the alcohol) and do shots of it every couple of hours. This cocktail/mocktail can easily be served with brunch or lunch and for those who need some nutritional assistance at the end of a busy day: it's the perfect happy hour drink. Don't be intimidated to make your own spinach juice. It's super easy and will give this drink live enzymes, which make it extra special and healthy for you. I add some spirulina to the coconut sugar for color and additional nutrition.

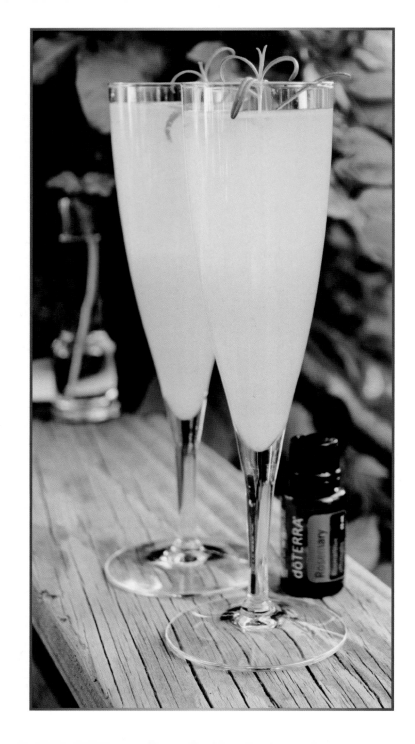

ROSEMARY INFUSED BELLINI

1 ounce rosemary-infused peach nectar

finish with prosecco

garnish with a rosemary sprig

Add rosemary-infused peach nectar to a champagne flute and top with prosecco.

PRIMARY BENEFITS

- supports healthy digestion
- supports healthy respiratory function
- helps to reduce tension and fatigue

ROSEMARY ESSENTIAL OIL

Rosemary is an aromatic, evergreen shrub whose leaves are frequently used to flavor foods such as stuffing, pork, roast lamb, chicken, and turkey. Along with its culinary applications, Rosemary has many benefits. Rosemary supports healthy digestion and internal organ function. Long revered by experts, Rosemary was considered sacred by the ancient Greek, Roman, Egyptian, and Hebrew cultures. Rosemary's herbaceous and energizing scent is frequently used in aromatherapy. Taken internally, it helps to reduce nervous tension and occasional fatigue.

NOTES FROM JULEZ

I have been mixing this delightful cocktail up for over a decade. Rosemary is a counterpart to lemon in that it aids the body in detoxification. What I love about this cocktail/ mocktail is its simplicity — it's really just a Bellini with a little herbal pizazz. It feels good in the body and makes the perfect addition to any brunch. Replace the prosecco with fizzy water to make it a mocktail. Serve it at brunch with a glass of water with a couple of drops of dōTERRA® lemon essential oil added, and you are really providing anyone with the ideal hangover remedy.

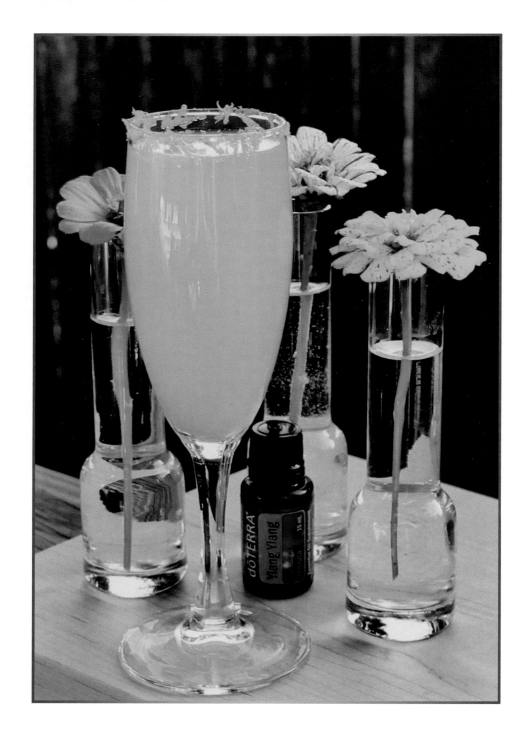

SEXY MANDARIN MIMOSA

1 ounce ylang ylang-infused mandarin juice
finish with champagne
garnish is optional

Add ylang ylang-infused mandarin juice to a champagne flute and top with Champagne.

YLANG YLANG ESSENTIAL OIL

Ylang Ylang essential oil is derived from the star-shaped flowers of the tropical Ylang Ylang tree and is used extensively in making perfumes and in aromatherapy. Similar to Jasmine, Ylang Ylang has been used for centuries in religious and wedding ceremonies. In aromatherapy, Ylang Ylang is used to lessen tension and stress and to promote a positive outlook. Ylang Ylang is frequently used in luxurious hair and skin products for its scent and nourishing and protective properties. Taken internally, Ylang Ylang provides antioxidant support.

NOTES FROM JULEZ

I have to say that the name of this cocktail is truly suiting. Ylang Ylang is a very sensual flower and its aromatic fragrance is intoxicating. What I love about this cocktail/mocktail is that it's a conversation piece. It's impossible to sip on this and not have something to say about it — it's that unique. It goes well with any brunch, and works for any special occasion. Replace the Champagne with fizzy water to make it a mocktail. It's tempting to replace the mandarin juice with orange juice, but I will say that it's not the same. Mandarin has more of an exotic flavor profile and Ylang Ylang beckons for something beyond your average orange. Trust me.

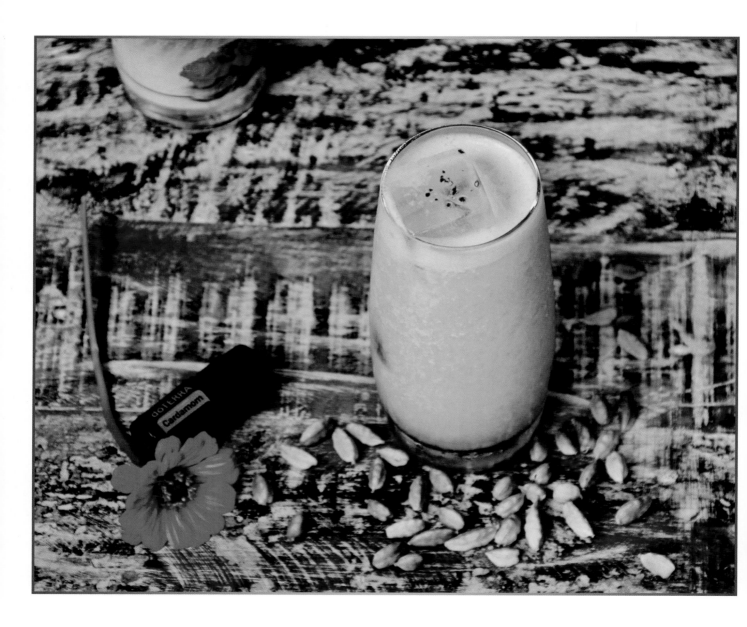

MANGO LASSÉ

2 ounces light rum

2 ounces mango juice

3 ounces of coconut milk or almond milk

1 teaspoon rose water

1 drop dōTERRA® cardamom essential oil

garnish with a pinch of cardamom on top

Fill shaker with ice. Layer ingredients in shaker, shake well and serve over ice in any tall glass.

CARDAMOM ESSENTIAL OIL

A close relative to Ginger, Cardamom is known as an expensive cooking spice and for being beneficial to the digestive system in a variety of ways. Cardamom is commonly used internally to help soothe occasional stomach discomfort. Its distinct scent can promote a positive mood. Ingested Cardamom also has profound effects on the respiratory system due to its high 1,8-cineole content, which promotes clear breathing and respiratory health. Native to Southeast Asia, Cardamom is added to traditional Indian sweets and teas for its cool, minty aroma and flavor. dōTERRA® Cardamom essential oil is extracted from Cardamom seeds grown in Guatemala, using our strict CPTG® testing standards. Through a collaborative and responsible sourcing arrangement, we are able to have a significant impact on the lives of local partners, ensuring that these farming communities enjoy improved livelihoods.

PRIMARY BENEFITS

- helps maintain gastrointestinal health
- promotes clear breathing
- promotes overall respiratory health

NOTES FROM JULEZ

A Mango Lassi is a traditional Indian drink made from different ingredients than this, but this is my take on it. I always loved the flavors and thought it would make a nice cocktail — and it does. It also makes an amazing mocktail, so feel free to leave out the rum. I jokingly call it a Lassé because the addition of rose water is so beautiful and feminine — it somehow feels French to me. Hence the name Mango Lassé. What I love about this cocktail/mocktail is that it has a bit of a tropical feel to it. It works well poolside or beachside and would also make a wonderful addition to a traditionally prepared Indian meal. Cardamom essential oil is an incredible aid for digestion and is deeply nurturing to the entire respiratory system.

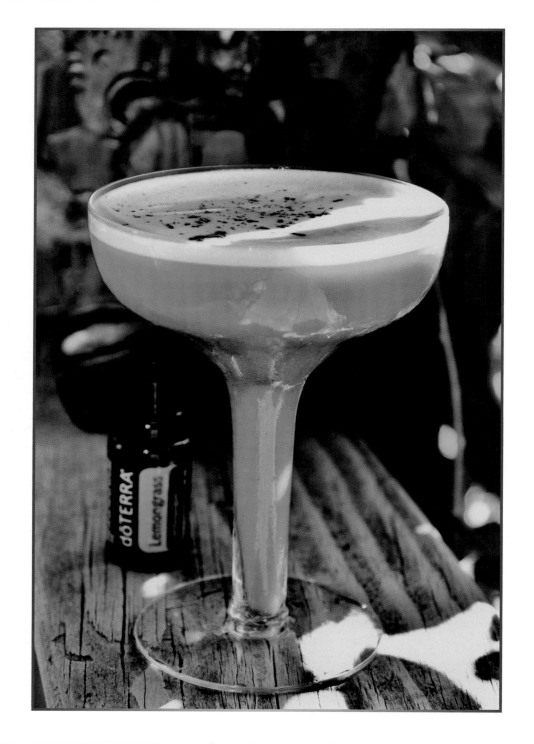

MATCHA LOVE

2 ounces light rum

5 ounces coconut or almond milk

1 teaspoon matcha powder

1 tablespoon lemongrass essential oil simple syrup

garish with a pinch of matcha powder on top

Fill shaker with ice. Layer ingredients in shaker, shake well and serve very cold in a coupe glass.

LEMONGRASS ESSENTIAL OIL

A tall, perennial plant, Lemongrass has a subtle citrus flavor and is used in Asian cuisine in soups, teas, and curries as well as with fish, poultry, beef, and seafood. In addition to its unique flavor, Lemongrass essential oil promotes healthy digestion and acts as an overall tonic to the body's systems when ingested. It's also purifying and toning to the skin, and is frequently used in skin care products for these benefits. Lemongrass is an ideal oil to use in massage therapy. Lemongrass has a pungent, herbaceous aroma that can heighten awareness and promote a positive outlook.

PRIMARY BENEFITS

- promotes a healthy outlook
- overall tonic for the body
- helps with circulation and digestion

NOTES FROM JULEZ

This is a really rockin' cocktail and is equally delicious as a mocktail. It can easily be served over ice if straight up isn't your jam. What I love about this cocktail/mocktail is that it's like an espresso martini replacement. Matcha green tea has a little bit of natural caffeine, but it also has a number of health benefits: it's high in antioxidants, boosts memory, enhances concentration, enhances the immune system and does loads of other amazing things for the body. The lemongrass goes nicely with the matcha and makes it a very uplifting experience. As a mocktail, this is great any time of the day and can even be served warm. As a cocktail, I like it as an after-work/before I go out on the town drink since the matcha can be a little stimulating and will give you a nice natural energy boost after a long day.

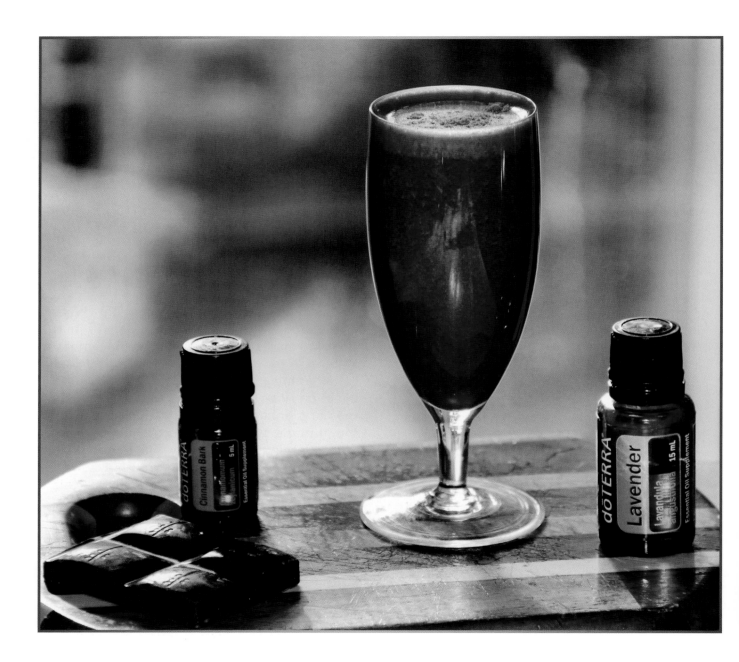

CACAO DREAMZ

1 cup almond milk or coconut milk

1 heaping tablespoon raw cacao powder

1 tablespoon honey or maple syrup

1 pinch of cayenne powder

1 pinch of Himalayan salt

1 drop dōTERRA® cinnamon essential oil

1 drop dōTERRA® lavender essential oil

garnish with a pinch of cinnamon powder

Place chosen milk in a saucepan. Add cacao powder and whisk over low heat. Once fully mixed add the honey, cayenne and Himalayan salt. Continue to whisk over low heat. Once the beverage is hot, turn the stovetop off and add the essential oils. Continue whisking for another minute. Serve warm in glass of choice. Pinch cinnamon on top. Please be mindful that cinnamon essential oil is very caustic. If any gets on your hands, refrain from touching face and immediately rub hands in fractionated coconut oil, or any other oil to dilute - don't use water.

LAVENDER ESSENTIAL OIL

Read about Lavender Essential Oil on page 41

CINNAMON ESSENTIAL OIL

Cinnamon is derived from a tropical, evergreen tree that grows up to 45 feet high and has highly fragrant bark, leaves, and flowers. Extracted from bark, Cinnamon oil supports healthy metabolic function and helps maintain a healthy immune system when needed most. Due to its high content of cinnamaldehyde, Cinnamon should be diluted with dōTERRA® Fractionated Coconut Oil when applied to the skin and only one to two drops are needed for internal benefits. Cinnamon has a long history of culinary uses, adding spice to desserts, entrees, and hot drinks.

PRIMARY BENEFITS

- supports healthy metabolic function
- maintains a healthy immune system
- long used to flavor food and enhance drinks

NOTES FROM JULEZ

I adore this elixir. It's a true expression of my alchemy and a gift to the soul. Cacao is such a beautiful, divine and ancient ingredient. It's food for the heart and spirit. There are so many things I could share about this wonderful delicacy but I sense you already know and have your own personal love with cacao. The cinnamon and lavender dance together to create spicy aromatic music in your mouth. This elixir is decadent and also has so many beneficial properties for your body. Sip it as a nightcap, make it dessert, serve it to those you love and they will love you for it.

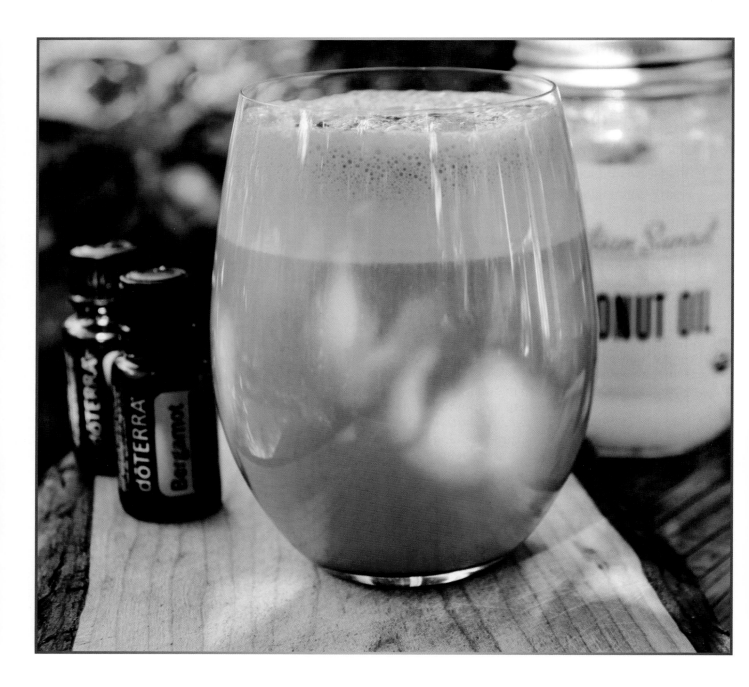

ESSENTIAL GOLDEN MILK

2 cups almond milk or coconut milk

1 tablespoon extra virgin coconut oil

1 tablespoon turmeric

1-2 tablespoons honey

1 drop dōTERRA® black pepper essential oil

1 drop dōTERRA® ginger essential oil

1 drop dōTERRA® bergamot essential oil

garnish with a pinch of cinnamon

Place chosen milk in a saucepan. Add turmeric and whisk over low heat. Once fully mixed, add the coconut oil and honey. Continue to whisk over low heat. Once the beverage is hot, turn the stovetop off and add the essential oils. Continue whisking for another minute. Serve warm in glass of choice. Pinch cinnamon on top. Serves 2-4 people you love.

GINGER ESSENTIAL OIL

Read about Ginger Essential Oil on page 43.

BLACK PEPPER ESSENTIAL OIL

Read about Black Pepper Essential Oil on page 65.

BERGAMOT ESSENTIAL OIL

Bergamot is unique among citrus oils due to its ability to be both uplifting and calming, making it ideal to help with anxious and sad feelings. It is also purifying and cleansing for the skin while having a calming effect.

PRIMARY BENEFITS

- calming and soothing aroma
- provides skin purifying benefits
- reduces feelings of stress

NOTES FROM JULEZ

Golden milk is a classic and timeless Ayurvedic elixir. Turmeric is loaded with curcumin, a polyphenol known for its ability to assist the body with inflammation, digestion and a variety of other ailments that tax our immune system. It's commonly made with ginger and black pepper, so the use of those two essential oils preserves this elixirs medicinal tapestry. I have also added bergamot essential oil as an aromatic enhancement and additional element to support overall well-being. What I love about this elixir is the way it makes me feel. It's served warm, so it feels great on a cold day or on a chilly night. It's wonderful to sip before bedtime. Adding this elixir to your daily health regime will assist you in a multitude of ways. Essential Golden Milk makes a stunning presentation when served in a glass. Serve to your guests alongside any dessert or make it the star of dessert - it will satisfy everyone's sweet tooth, and give their body a big gift!

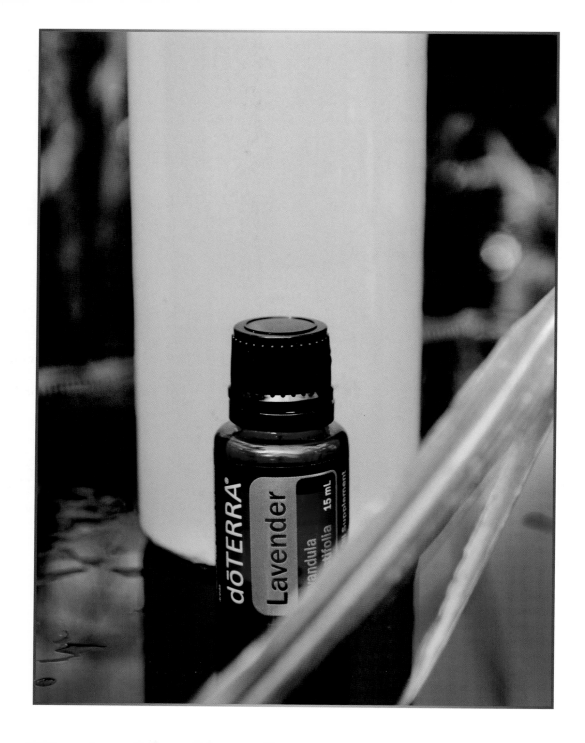

THE ESSENTIAL MIXOLOGIST KIT

- **Bergamot**
- **Black Pepper**
- **Cinnamon**
- **Cardamom**
- **Cilantro**
- **Ginger**
- **Grapefruit**
- **Lavender**
- **Lemon**

- **Lemongrass**
- **Lime**
- **On Guard® Blend**
- **Rosemary**
- **Tangerine**
- **Spearmint**
- **Wild Orange**
- **Yang Ylang**

dōTERRA® is a wonderful choice for all of your essential oil needs. We also carry many other essential oil enhanced wellness products. If you don't already have a dōTERRA® account, please feel free to contact me and we will set you up. If someone has been speaking with you already about dōTERRA®, please honor that relationship and contact them for guidance on getting started.

There is also an incredible business opportunity for those who are passionate about health & wellness and enjoy helping others. We are always looking for new people to join our team and would be happy to connect with anyone who is genuinely interested in our business.

For more information please visit

www.essentialmixologist.com

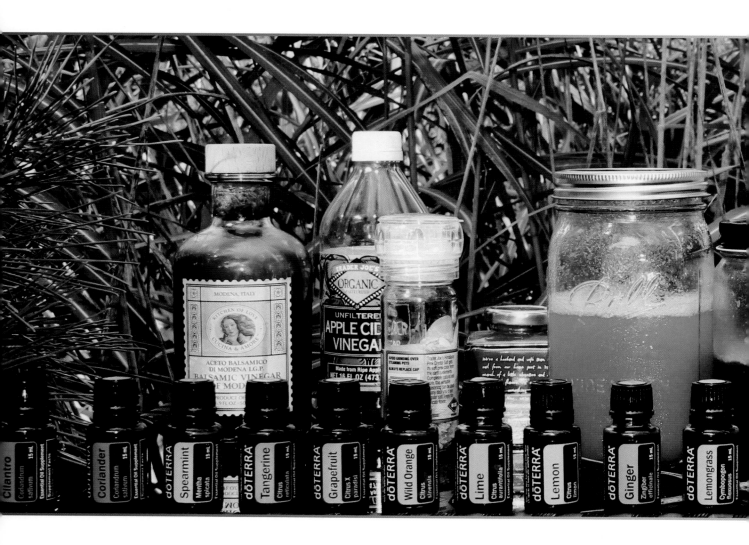

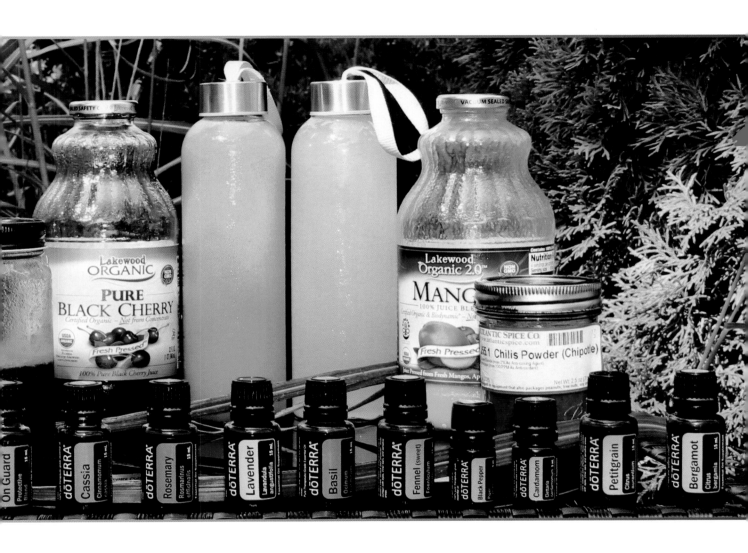

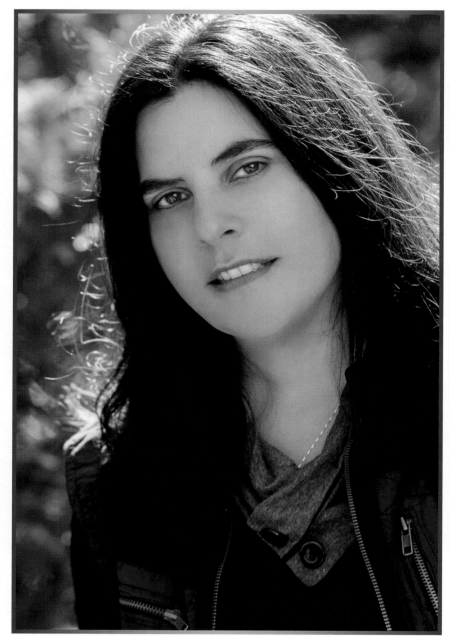

Photo by Gregg Peterson